# THE FOOT AND ITS COVERING.

PLATE 1.

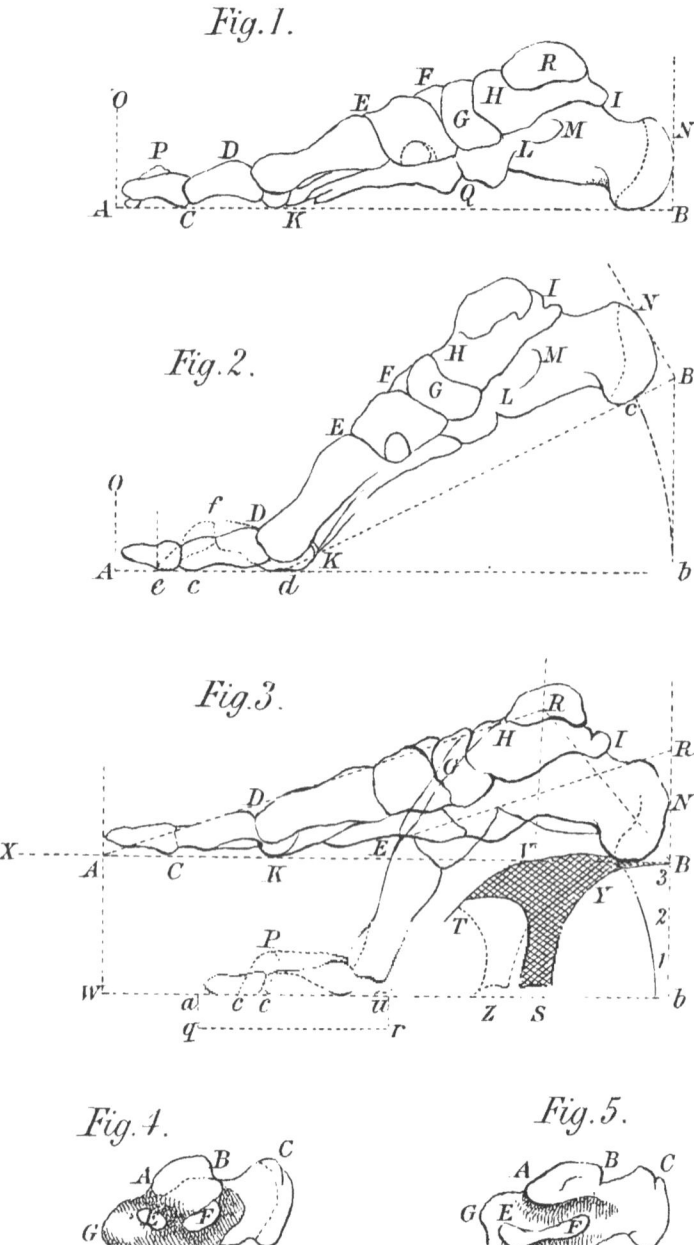

# The Foot

## AND

## ITS COVERING,

### WITH

### DR. CAMPER'S WORK "ON THE BEST FORM OF SHOE,"

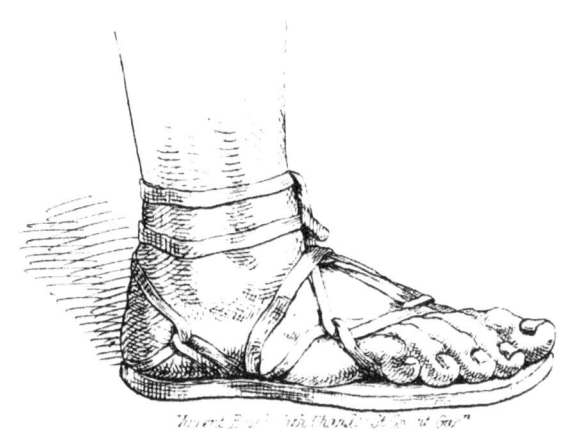

## BY JAMES DOWIE.

# A History of Shoemaking

Shoemaking, at its simplest, is the process of making footwear. Whilst the art has now been largely superseded by mass-volume industrial production, for most of history, making shoes was an individual, artisanal affair. 'Shoemakers' or 'cordwainers' (cobblers being those who repair shoes) produce a range of footwear items, including shoes, boots, sandals, clogs and moccasins – from a vast array of materials.

When people started wearing shoes, there were only three main types: open sandals, covered sandals and clog-like footwear. The most basic foot protection, used since ancient times in the Mediterranean area, was the sandal, which consisted of a protective sole, attached to the foot with leather thongs. Similar footwear worn in the Far East was made from plaited grass or palm fronds. In climates that required a full foot covering, a single piece of untanned hide was laced with a thong, providing full protection for the foot, thus forming a complete covering. These were the main two types of footwear, produced all over the globe. The production of wooden shoes was mainly limited to medieval Europe however – made from a single piece of wood, roughly shaped to fit the foot.

A variant of this early European shoe was the clog, which were wooden soles to which a leather upper was attached. The sole and heel were generally made from one piece of maple or ash two inches thick, and a little longer and broader than the desired size of shoe. The outer side of the sole and heel was fashioned with a long chisel-edged implement, called the clogger's knife or stock; while a second implement, called the groover, made a groove around the side of the sole. With the use of a 'hollower', the inner sole's contours were adapted to the shape of the foot. In even colder climates, such designs were adapted with furs wrapped around the feet, and then sandals wrapped over them. The Romans used such footwear to great effect whilst fighting in Northern Europe, and the native Indians developed similar variants with their ubiquitous moccasin.

By the 1600s, leather shoes came in two main types. 'Turn shoes' consisted of one thin flexible sole, which was sewed to the upper while outside in and turned over when completed. This type was used for making slippers and similar shoes. The second type united the upper with an insole, which was subsequently attached to an out-sole with a raised heel. This was the main variety, and was used for most footwear, including standard shoes and riding boots.

Shoemaking became more commercialized in the mid-eighteenth century, as it expanded as a cottage industry. Large warehouses began to stock footwear made by many small manufacturers from the area. Until the nineteenth century, shoemaking was largely a traditional handicraft, but by the century's end, the process had been almost completely mechanized, with production occurring in large factories. Despite the obvious economic gains of mass-production, the factory system produced shoes without the individual differentiation that the traditional shoemaker was able to provide.

The first steps towards mechanisation were taken during the Napoleonic Wars by the English engineer, Marc Brunel. He developed machinery for the mass-production of boots for the soldiers of the British Army. In 1812 he devised a scheme for making nailed-boot-making machinery that automatically fastened soles to uppers by means of metallic pins or nails. With the support of the Duke of York, the shoes were manufactured, and, due to their strength, cheapness, and durability, were introduced for the use of the army. In the same year, the use of screws and staples was patented by Richard Woodman. However, when the war ended in 1815, manual labour became much cheaper again, and the demand for military equipment subsided. As a consequence, Brunel's system was no longer profitable and it soon ceased business.

Similar exigencies at the time of the Crimean War stimulated a renewed interest in methods of mechanization and mass-production, which proved longer lasting. A shoemaker in Leicester, Tomas Crick, patented the design for a riveting machine in 1853. He also introduced the use of steam-powered rolling-machines for hardening leather and cutting-machines, in the mid-1850s. Another important factor in shoemaking's mechanization, was the introduction of the sewing machine in 1846 – a development which revolutionised so many aspects of clothes, footwear and domestic production.

By the late 1850s, the industry was beginning to shift towards the modern factory, mainly in the US and areas of England. A shoe stitching machine was invented by the American Lyman Blake in 1856 and perfected by 1864.

Entering in to partnership with Gordon McKay, his device became known as the McKay stitching machine and was quickly adopted by manufacturers throughout New England. As bottlenecks opened up in the production line due to these innovations, more and more of the manufacturing stages, such as pegging and finishing, became automated. By the 1890s, the process of mechanisation was largely complete.

Traditional shoemakers still exist today, especially in poorer parts of the world, and do continue to create custom shoes. In more economically developed countries however, it is a dying craft. Despite this, the shoemaking profession makes a number of appearances in popular culture, such as in stories about shoemaker's elves (written by the Brothers Grimm in 1806), and the old proverb that 'the shoemaker's children go barefoot.' Chefs and cooks sometimes use the term 'shoemaker' as an insult to others who have prepared sub-standard food, possibly by overcooking, implying that the chef in question has made his or her food as tough as shoe leather or hard leather shoe soles. Similarly, reflecting the trade's humble beginnings, to 'cobble' can mean not only to make or mend shoes, but 'to put together clumsily; or, to bungle.'

As is evident from this short introduction, 'shoemaking' has a long and varied history, starting from a simple means of providing basic respite from the elements, to a fully mechanised and modern, global trade. It is able to provide a fascinating insight not only into fashion, but society, culture and climate more generally. We hope the reader enjoys this book.

# THE FOOT AND ITS COVERING;

COMPRISING

A FULL TRANSLATION OF DR. CAMPER'S WORK

ON

"THE BEST FORM OF SHOE."

BY JAMES DOWIE.

"I hold every man a debtor to his profession; from the which, as men of course doe seeke to receive countenance and profit, so ought they of duty to endeavour themselves, by way of amends, to be a help and an ornament thereunto."—BACON.

TO

# SIR BENJAMIN COLLINS BRODIE, BART.,

President of the Royal Society,

SERJEANT-SURGEON TO THE QUEEN.

SIR,

 THE elevated position which you hold in that distinguished Society, ever foremost in the investigation of the great laws of Nature ; the prominent place which, during a long life, you have devoted to mitigate the sufferings of mankind, physically and socially ; and the kind condescension which you have shown in patronizing even the humblest efforts in the cause of progress, (as experienced by myself on my arrival in London more than twenty years ago), have encouraged me to inscribe this humble volume to you, in grateful testimony and esteem of your kind permission.

     By your obliged

       And very humble servant,

         JAMES DOWIE.

# GENERAL PREFACE.

This Work is intended as a popular introduction to the study of the Human Foot and its Covering, from a Shoemaker's point of view. Having had the misfortune to lose both my parents before I had reached my twelfth year, my guardians, in 1815, apprenticed me to the trade of a shoemaker. In 1830, I had the pleasure to receive from a medical friend, in token of his esteem, a copy of Paley's works. I was then assiduously pursuing business on my own account in my native city, Edinburgh, to the satisfaction of those who had hitherto been my guardians. When I received my friend's gift—one which I shall never forget, because it shed a gleam of new light on my labours, for Paley's chapter on "The Faculty of Standing" so thoroughly convinced me how much more physiological anatomy had to do with the manufacture of boots and shoes than I had previously imagined, that I lost no time in acquiring all the information I could on the subject. The progress I thus made in this important branch of science I followed up by a lengthened experimental inquiry relative to the introduction of elastic materials into the soles and uppers of boots and shoes to accommodate them to the functions of the foot.

Edinburgh, even at that time, afforded many facilities for acquiring information of the kind I was in search of. Indeed, no sooner had I enunciated my proposition of an elastic principle in the clothing of the foot, than it was appreciated by the medical profession; and Dr. Monro, Sir George Ballingall, and Dr. Thomson had the kindness to grant me permission to attend their lectures on Anatomy, Military Surgery, and Physiology. These invitations I thankfully accepted, profiting to the best of my humble ability by everything they respectively taught in the direction in which I was seeking for information.

For a Shoemaker to be aware that there is a distinguishable difference between his foot and his last, will not be considered beyond his sphere of knowledge. But the amount of difference that does exist between the two is a very different thing. Before I acquired the information referred to, I certainly had no conception that the difference was so great as it is; and when I began to instruct my workmen, some twenty-six in number, in the manufacture of elastic boots and shoes, more than one of them expressed their astonishment to hear that there was any difference at all, or that it was such as to require elasticated leather, and, above all, that it was necessary to take them from their own houses to work under my own immediate superintendence.

Having myself received much benefit from studying the anatomical specimens in the Surgeons' Hall, it occurred to me that a visit of my men to that place would put things right. Accordingly, I procured tickets of admission for them, and the result was a complete revolution in the men's minds; some who had hastily left my work regretting it afterwards.

It was not the amount of information my men received by a single visit to the Surgeons' Hall that produced the favourable change in their minds, but the stimulus which that visit gave to the investigation of their own feet, and the nature of the covering the human foot required. Although they had been daily employed in making boots and shoes, their attention had never before been turned to the difference that existed between the lasts upon which boots and shoes were made, and the feet upon which they were to be worn. They were familiar with the former, went to the Surgeons' Hall to make themselves acquainted with the internal structure of the latter, and returned to their work with minds divested of former prejudices, and thus much the wiser to begin the world again.

My object in presenting this little volume to the

public is something similar to what I had in view when I sent my men to the Surgeons' Hall. I knew, for example, that on their return home from that place they would examine their own feet from an anatomical point of view, and the nature of the covering which their mechanical functions required; and this is just what I hope my little work will induce its readers to do. There is, perhaps, no part of our clothing that is more subject to criticism than our boots and shoes, and no member of the body that gives occasion to more consideration than the foot. Now, in such cases, are our views always correct? Do we examine the latter and criticize the former as we ought to do, considering the dependence of our general health upon the relation that exists between them? It was by the handling and examination of my own feet, on reading Paley, &c., I discovered that the rule I had been taught relative to measuring the foot and allowing a certain uniform increase of length to the last, was erroneous, and that by following this rule I was doing injustice to myself, my profession, and my customers; and without saying a word here in favour of the practice I now pursue relative to measurement, I can have no hesitation in condemning the one I previously followed, and in recommending to the dispassionate consideration of the reader my reasons for doing so, which will be found in the body of the work.

In the British Museum and other libraries of the

metropolis, German and French editions of Dr Camper's essay on the best form of shoe are to be seen. It was a Dr. Staunton, of ——, in Ireland, who, in calling for a copy of my former paper on the subject of shoes, first drew my attention to Camper's work; but not being acquainted with foreign languages, I could not profit by the German copy which I first saw. The title and drawings, however, made me very anxious to get possession of a copy, for the purpose of translation; but after a fruitless search of several years, in this country and on the continent of Europe, I finally thought of employing a translator and an artist to procure a translation, with a copy of the drawings, from the library of the British Museum.

Accidentally the artist I employed mentioned the circumstance to a brother artist—a customer of mine, and very intimate friend—who had a French copy of Dr. Camper's work, and he at once made me a present of it. Having thus obtained a French copy, I was anxious to give a translation of it, and on showing the work to a medical friend, an excellent French scholar, he kindly supplied what I now have the pleasure of laying before my readers—an English edition of this invaluable work.

In the portion of the following work which is mine, I have discussed the several topics in the order in which they have always engaged and continue to occupy my own attention as a Shoemaker, under the conviction that this will be found generally advantageous. The subject is one of such voluminous dimensions, that I have experienced no little difficulty in confining it within the limited number of pages prescribed for it; and if I have appropriated more space to one chapter and less to another than I might have done, it is because I think the peculiar merits of the respective topics and their state of progress required such treatment. For the cursory manner in which many interesting sections are handled, I shall, no doubt, have to plead an exceptional brevity to many of my readers.

My two former papers on this subject, read before the Royal Scottish Society of Arts (the one in 1835 and the other in 1839), having received the highest marks of approbation bestowed upon the like, not only by its members, but also by the engineers and medical profession of London, as well as of Edinburgh, gave me every encouragement to proceed with the present work. At the same time, my elasticated leather met with no little opposition. This is not to be wondered at, when it is seen that my proposition is diametrically opposed to the rigid-soled system generally followed; while many who wished well to the cause I had at heart, accused me of being too enthusiastic in my advocacy of the elastic principle in the manufacture of boots and shoes. The opposition I have met with has doubtless been further increased by the earnestness with which I have all along pressed my proposition upon the attention of the Government.

The warm support it met with from many distinguished military officers of the higher rank, however, as well as from members of both branches of the legislature, seemed to justify me in this course. But then the antiquated state of the clothing department of the public service, especially in reference to boots and shoes, as the number of "Blue Books" that have appeared on the subject testifies, stood in my way; I hope, however, that the present work will vindicate me, and those who have supported me, from all adverse charges. Indeed, when such men as Sir George Ballingall, professor of military surgery, in lecturing on military foot-dress, advocated the elastic principle introduced by me, I should have looked upon myself as a "*deserter*," had I turned my back upon the cause of progress in the shoeing of the British soldier.

No doubt my proposition involves a revolution in the manufacture of boots and shoes, and, to a certain extent, in the materials of which they are made; but those who will take the trouble to study the anatomical structure of their own feet, and the nature of the covering they require, will be constrained to wish with the author a speedy consummation to such an event. In consequence of the rapid progress which this revolution is now making, I have said less upon the handicraft department of my subject than otherwise I should have done. .As agriculturists, engineers, and others, in every branch of science and industry, are laying before the public in books the rudiments of their respective professions, with a view to progress—I in like manner have ventured, as a humble Shoemaker, to publish an elementary work on the Human Foot and its Covering, in the hope of contributing in some small degree to the advancement of that branch of industry with which I am connected.

JAMES DOWIE.

455, Strand, London.

# CONTENTS.

|  | Page |
|---|---|
| GENERAL PREFACE | vii |

## Part the First.

|  | |
|---|---|
| PREFACE TO "CAMPER ON THE BEST FORM OF SHOE" | xxvii |
| INTRODUCTION | 1 |

### CHAPTER I.
| THE FOOT | 9 |
|---|---|

### CHAPTER II.
| THE BONES OF THE FOOT | 13 |
|---|---|

### CHAPTER III.
| THE SOLE OF THE FOOT | 21 |
|---|---|

### CHAPTER IV.
| UPON WALKING | 25 |
|---|---|

### CHAPTER V.
| SHOES AND BOOTS | 30 |
|---|---|

### CHAPTER VI.
| OF THE BEST SHAPE OF A SHOE | 35 |
|---|---|

### CHAPTER VII.
| OF THE INCONVENIENCES OCCASIONED BY ILL-MADE SHOES, AND THEIR REMEDIES | 38 |
|---|---|

## Part the Second.

### CHAPTER I.

#### INTRODUCTION.

Dr. Camper's Essay; notice of — Comparison between Dr. Camper's and Dowie's Paper before the Royal Scottish Society of Arts—Principal difference; elasticated leather—Elastic material the real object sought by Dr. Camper—Elongation of the Foot under pressure, treated more fully by Dowie's paper—Dowie's paper got up to procure Scottish Society of Arts' patronage—Is wanting in many respects—Demand for the present work—His duty in reply—Apology for imperfections and anxiety to discharge his duty—Customer and shoemaker equally interested in progress—Grand consideration; welfare of Foot generally neglected—Practice, with science, the best rule—Twofold division of the work, Foot and Covering.—*Page* 46—53.

### CHAPTER II.

#### EXTERNAL ANATOMY OF THE FOOT, ETC.

No two feet alike—A proper Fit a proper covering—What is the nature of the covering?—Ever-varying form of the Foot — Measurement consequently different — Differences arise from mechanical functions in progression—Dr. Camper's view, anatomical; Author's mechanical—Foot and leg system of leverage—Almost every bone of Foot a lever—The movements of walking described—The best example everybody's own case in walking—Elongation of Foot—Of a twofold character—Elongation on the principles of a carriage spring—Momentum added to weight of body in walking increases flattening—Second kind of elongation at the root of toes—When toes turned up; elongation in front — When toes rest on ground; elongation backwards—Elongation backwards compensated in part—Bones of Foot form a double arch—Lateral and longitudinal expansion forwards—Increases strength of Foot—Longitudinal expansion greatest in long, high instep, and *vice versâ*—Lateral expansion greatest in high-arched broad feet, and *vice versâ*—Flattening of the arch in front in walking; great going up-hill—Arch flattens at heel in going down-hill—Going downstairs test of strength of Foot—Form and position of great toe—Different forms of the great toe—Thickness at the point, two extremes and a mean given—Length of great toe, two extremes and a mean given—Form of the Foot in front; Dr. Camper quoted—Example of broad flat Foot, first extreme—Narrow Foot, second extreme—Well-formed Foot, middle life, infancy, and old age, peculiarities of—Special notice of dome-shaped arch of Foot; its GREAT CREATOR'S work — Diversities of longitudinal and lateral expansion—High instep narrow above, first extreme —Nearly flat Foot, flat above, second extreme—Medium arch, mean between two extremes—Projection of heelbone; in Indians; difference in different individuals—Diversity of ankle; ankle joint an important fulcrum—Astragalus and its influence in position of ankle and heelbone—Muscles and foot-tackle must be in trim.—*Page* 54—72.

## CHAPTER III.

### PHYSICAL WELL-BEING OF THE FOOT.

Introduction—Foot and its influence on general health—Not sufficiently attended to—Indifference to health unpardonable —Reason assigned for such unsettled questions in science— Waste given off between toes—Greatest with bad shoeing and exercise—Exercise yet essential to health—No sort of material but muscle could stand what it does in long journeys —External anatomy the shoemaker's question, for if outside is right so will the inside of Foot—Exercise—Freedom of function in shoe—As when barefoot—Consequences when otherwise—Contracts disease—Various diseases, two classes—When a customer orders first let the health of his Foot be first question—Cultivation of health—Normal state improved—Rope-dancers, &c.—Means which improve health of Foot improve general health—Proof by grasping leg, thighs, &c.—Paley quoted—Suspension of action of one part increases the strain upon others, rendering walking a painful wasting instead of a blessing—Walking and its importance generally considered; metropolis, &c.—Physiological anatomists everywhere pointing to Foot as foundation of health—Present sanitary and volunteer movements and their tendency—The individual question the most important, because everybody's question.—*Page* 73—84.

## CHAPTER IV.

### INQUIRY INTO THE NATURE OF THE COVERING OF THE FOOT, ETC.

Introduction to chapter—Elasticity — Expansibility of Foot requires the same of shoe—Negative proof, rocking lever—Wooden leg—Horse and donkey shoes—Absurdity of rigid shoes, &c.—Requirement of Foot different at different ages—Infancy—Growing Foot easily injured, but sound in good shoes—Exercise and action of light to stimulate growth—A proper covering necessary to insure exercise—Shoemaker has to provide for increase of size as well as the tender structure of Foot—Author's anxiety for the welfare of the Foot in childhood—Foot from five to fourteen, peculiarities—Foot from fourteen to twenty, peculiarities—Youth's responsibility—Fashion — Manhood and old age — Clerks, &c.—Merchants—Building-trades, millers, &c.—Farmers, sportsmen, &c.—Soldiers—Sailors—Summer, winter, &c.—*Page* 85—95.

CONTENTS. xix

## CHAPTER V.

#### MEASUREMENT.—STOCKING AND LAST.

Introduction — Diagram showing mode of measuring — The difference of length between rule and atlas—Elongation of Foot—Provision made for extremes — Elongation at the waist of boot or shoe—Growing Foot at toe, &c.—Second kind of elongation, provision for—Elastic waist, provision for first kind—Extra length at toe for second kind—The proper length more a matter of judgment than measurement—Measurement of toes—Atlas necessary—Importance of a proper fit for the toes—Girth not sufficient—Main points, four—Thickness, position, and curvature the chief—Great toe and little toe, protection for—Girths of metatarsus and tarsus—Provision for heel—Instep on line with leg—Increases arch—Going over the sole inside and outside, cause of—Both feet to be measured—Review of measurement; conclusion—How does the stocking fit? not well — The Foot in childhood injured—Toes afterwards grow worse and worse—Ought not the stocking to have toes?—Toed stocking increases breath of Foot — The last measurement and classification — Regular customer; last and measurement booked together — First measurement; new last often—Rule; every Foot should have its own last—On the making of lasts; every one should have a boot-tree of his own.—*Page* 96—111.

## CHAPTER VI.

#### ON RAW MATERIALS.

Introduction—Boots and shoes; bulk of, made of leather—How quality of leather is being deteriorated—Rage for cheap boots; cause of splitting hides, &c. — Tanned, curried, and tawed leathers; variety of—Principal defects of leather—Leather, its primitive character; improvement, march of—

Manufactured fabrics, progress of—Principles involved, two-fold—Spirit of progress at work; must triumph.—*Page* 112—116.

## CHAPTER VII.

#### ON THE CONSTRUCTION OF BOOTS AND SHOES.

Introductory remarks—Application of measurement; different kind of boots; principles involved—Difference between back, belly, and flank of hides; economy of material, cutting, making, trade of in such points separately—Finishing for the last involves skill—Skill in putting uppers on the last—Uppers should be stretched equally—General properties of sole—Thin sole better than a thick one; reason why—Sole must elongate—Cannot be cut out of ordinary sole leather; elasticated material at waist—Print of the sole of the Foot—Relationship between it; form of sole—Right and left sole; its origin—Object of right and left soles—Clothing of instep; differences of different feet—Sewing machinery used in certain customer-work; uppers—Soles sewed to uppers; rivetting, &c.—Province of fashion must not injure Foot—Objectionable notions of; subject requires ventilation.—*Page* 117—124.

## CHAPTER VIII.

#### ON THE CONSTRUCTION OF THE BOOTS AND SHOES NOW GENERALLY WORN, AND THEIR ADAPTATION TO THE FOOT.

Introductory remarks—Strong lacing-boot of labourer; general description of—Importance of the general question the boot as it is and as it should be—Example of laced boot on pedestrians; three miles to one—Sir Charles Bell quoted in his remarkable extracts—Extra expenditure of muscular force—Stilts *v.* no stilts—Lacing-boot; "spring of the last;" rocking lever—Light step of trained pedestrians and economy of muscular force—Effects of. lacing-boot on rising generation—Example two, fashionable toes—Facts v. fashionable toes—Wedging of the toes, without parallel in history of dress—Solution of the problem in deformed toes and boots—Deformity a gradual process—Deformity of Foot gives rise to change of shoe—Case of infancy and youth; process of malformation—Toes wedged sideways and between soles and uppers—Fashionable heels; Dr. Camper quoted—Additional examples advanced—Example 1, standing on an incline plane—Example 2, high heels worse than stilts—Example 3, fashionable waist and high heels force up key-stone—Concluding remarks. —*Page* 125—142.

## CHAPTER IX.

### ON WELLINGTONS AND BLUCHERS.

Introduction—Object of chapter, improvement—Details reciprocally applicable, soldier's foot-dress a public question—Figs. 1, 2, 3, army boots—Measurement—Straight sole similar to Dr. Camper's—Fleshy part of great toe may be flattened—The questions at issue relating to the great toe—Great toe wedged only so far in the middle of toe of boot—Broad toe worse than narrow; great toe in the middle of boot—Drawing of deformed Foot, &c.—Drs. Holden and Paley quoted relating to natural form of toes—On the waist and level sole of the foot outside—The manner the lateral arch is injured; sole levelled and flat foot; Police and other cases—When curved waist is reduced, that of the sole is increased—Increasing the spring of the last and reducing the radius—Robin Hood's arrow *v.* "Spring of the last"—Propositions necessary for consideration—The wheel theory; absurdity of—Childish toys; argument involved—The Foot an elastic, self-elongating lever—Pedestrian *v.* soldier—Threefold character of elongating lever—Two extremes and mean explained—Right-angled triangle, &c.—Lever elongated by muscular force—This elongation that produces uniform motion and level of the body—Elasticity of Foot more requisite when running—Example of soldier illustrated—*Modus operandi* of starting soldiers, centrifugal—Knapsack, &c. 60lbs.; centrifugal effects of—Exact rise and fall not known—Parallel case, steam-engine—Zigzag movements greater, explained—Lateral movements of the Foot destroyed—Deprived of these elasticity destroyed—Grinding of soles on the ground—Centre of gravity has to be brought more on one foot—Trained pedestrian centre of gravity moves in curved line—Much depends upon how boot fits; seven moulds only—Applicable to all ready-made work—Reason why—More attention to fashion than form of Foot—Summary of objections.—*Page* 143—167.

## CHAPTER X.

### ELASTICATED LEATHER—ITS OBJECT, VALUE, ETC.

Origin of elasticated leather—Experiments with India-rubber waist—Sir John Robinson's experiment and failure—Invention of elasticated leather—Its composition and manufacture—Different varieties of the fabric—Preparation of raw materials—Invention of elastic sandal tie—Strength and durability of elasticated leather—Stands difference of temperature—The elastic principle sound—Extent to which it is applicable.—*Page* 168—174.

## CHAPTER XI.

### ON INJURED FEET, ETC.

Introductory remarks—Injured feet restored to symmetry—Obstacles in the way of; process slow—Healthy constitutions; feet soon begin to recover—Practical examples—Arch of the Foot—In soldiers and police—Metropolitan police—Manner cure is effected—Case of crooked toes—Injured metatarsus—

CONTENTS. xxiii

How toes are injured ; also metatarsus—Reformatory process in both cases—Provision required in the covering.—*Page* 175—184.

## CHAPTER XII.

### ON TRADE SYSTEMS, ETC.

Introductory remarks—Boots to order ; ready-made ; pattern, &c.—Commercial values—Intrinsic values—Style—Reason of present defective style—Style not justifiable for the future—Comparative merits, &c.—Greater health of Foot greater durability of boot—Duty relative to cultivation ; Greek and Roman practices—Two important ends ; duties involved—Voice of public ; in favour of exercise—No attention to improve Foot ; singularity of—Prevention better than cure—Duty of parents and guardians—Duty of Government—Official mismanagement—Reasons for improvement—The British lion — Military experiments with elastic boots — Case of volunteers—Duty of shoemakers, last makers, &c.—Objections refuted.—*Page* 185—198.

## CHAPTER XIII.

### CONCLUSION.

Importance of the subject—Examples from Nature—Nature's instructive works—Reviews of measurement, &c.—Reviews of present construction of boots and shoes — Reviews of elasticated material — Concluding observations.—*Page* 199—204.

# PART I.

## ON THE BEST FORM OF SHOE.

### BY PETER CAMPER, M.D.,

PROFESSOR OF MEDICINE, SURGERY, AND ANATOMY, AT AMSTERDAM AND GRONINGEN.

Calceus pede major subvertit, minor urit.

The shoe too large, the foot will wring ;
Too small, 'twill corns and bunions bring.

# PREFACE TO "CAMPER ON THE BEST FORM OF SHOE."

This little treatise originated in a jest. I wished to prove to my pupils, who maintained that all subjects had been treated in writing until they were exhausted, that the most trifling matter, were it but a *shoe*, might become interesting if discussed by one able to speak with entire knowledge of both causes and results.

They did not believe that I should dare to make public such a work on such a subject. I accepted the challenge, and here it is.

But, joking apart, my reasonings upon the distressing consequences of the miserable manner in which we are at present shod are founded upon a long series of observations and reiterated experience. I can only hope that the victims of fashion may profit by my views, and that many fathers and mothers will be induced to avoid the infliction of much torture upon their children. If I can succeed in persuading them of this, I shall have accomplished my object.

I shall not say—

> Ridendo castigat mores,
> Jesting, your manners I were fain to mend;

but—

> Ridendo calceos corrigit,
> Jesting, to improve your foot-gear I intend.

# INTRODUCTION.

"Non multum abfuit, quin sutrinum quoque inventum à sapientibus diceret Posidonius."—SENECA.

IT is surprising that while mankind in all ages have bestowed the greatest attention upon the feet of horses, mules, oxen, and other animals of burthen or draught, they have entirely neglected those of their own species, abandoning them to the ignorance of workmen, who, in general, can only make a shoe upon routine principles, and according to the absurdities of fashion, or the depraved taste of the day. Thus, from our earliest infancy, shoes, as at present worn, serve but to deform the toes and cover the feet with corns, which not only render walking painful, but, in some cases, absolutely impossible. All this is caused by the ignorance of our shoemakers.

We bestow reasonable compassion upon the fate of the Chinese women, who dislocate their feet in obedience to the dictates of a barbarous custom, and yet we ourselves have submitted complacently for ages to tortures no less cruel. I say for ages:

C. Celsus, who lived before the Christian era, Paulus Ægineta, and Ætius, have described, with great precision, the diseases of the feet caused by ill-made shoes and sandals. It is evident that all the world did not imitate Socrates, who went barefoot.

The shoes and boots of our time are no better than those of the ancients. I know by experience the difficulty of obtaining easy ones. I have never met with such in London, and rarely in Paris; but at Amsterdam and Groningen I found several makers, grown grey in their business, who entered into my views when they saw the sad evidences of unwilling experience on my own feet; above all, however, and as having served me best, both in regard to ease in walking and excellence of the article, I have to commend a young master cordwainer of the Hague.

Experience and reflection soon led me to the conclusion that a shoe adapted to one town may not be so well suited to another. A shoe, for example, fitted for the Hague, is not so for Amsterdam, and is positively objectionable at Leeuwarden, at Groningen, and wherever the streets are paved with rolled pebbles, as nature presents them to us, and without being dressed and squared, as they are at Hamburg, Berlin, &c. Elsewhere the pavements are still worse, and there a certain habit is necessary to escape disagreeable inconveniences in walking.

I am confident, moreover, that even the best and most celebrated shoemakers have a defective method of taking the measure of the foot. My knowledge of anatomy shows me that the foot lengthens in walking, and becomes shorter when in repose. In consequence, the measure taken of the sole of the foot when in repose, according to ordinary routine, must produce a shoe too short for the same foot when it is in motion; and thus both the great toe and the heel must be pinched, and the joints of all the toes made to rise, and form eminences, the sole being of too unyielding a material to adapt itself to the necessities of the case. Experience has convinced me, also, that the heels of boots and shoes ought to be placed more forward upon the sole, so as to support the centre of gravity of the body. I remember that in my boyhood shoes were made with the toes slightly turned up. Our travelled youth introduced the Parisian fashion of wearing them very flat and shallow, and with excessively high heels. A general revolution in the fashion of our shoes ensued. I purchased shoes of this description for myself, without noticing the change, but was painfully made aware of it at the expense of my toes, which were bruised by contact with every stone that came in my way. The reason of this discomfort was an enigma to me until, the subject of shoes and shoemaking having occupied my mind, I discovered the cause of my martyrdom.

The principles of my researches are founded upon the anatomical theory of Borelli. They have convinced me of the importance of the subject, and induce me to believe that I may be of some service to my fellow-creatures, by enabling them to profit by my physical inquiries into the defects of a part of our attire with which we cannot dispense.

Men and women do not walk in the same manner, on account of the difference in the width of their hips; and children, again, move differently, in consequence of the shortness of their legs. Aged persons, whose heads (and frequently their bodies also) are bowed forward, are obliged to bend the knees to preserve their equilibrium,—the centre of gravity then falling necessarily more forward upon the instep.

Towards the end of pregnancy, moreover, the upper part of the female frame is thrown backwards, in order to maintain the centre of gravity; so that at this important period women bear greatly on the heel.

Ladies, old and young, in the upper walks of life, wear high and slender heels to their foot-gear; and to make the foot look smaller and neater, these heels are carried as far forward under the instep as possible. Misled by ridiculous vanity, our burgesses have also adopted this absurd fashion. Our peasantry are wiser, they providing themselves with shoes that give firmness to their gait and render walking easy.

Tall persons walk in a peculiar manner, and require, in consequence, shoes adapted to their step. Education has also considerable influence upon the shape of the foot: a gentleman always turns out his toes, while a peasant as invariably turns them in. The celebrated M. André has fully discussed this subject, in his "*Orthopédie,*" pp. 254, 255. It is incontestable that the proper position of the feet is to have them turned out, and that this attitude contributes to the stability of the body when erect; because with the two feet we then form a sort of triangle, which gives all the security of the tripod. It is with justice, therefore, that in the dancing school the position of the toes turned in is designated the false position. *Vide* "Dictionnaire Encyclopédique," vol. viii., Pl. I., figs. 9, 10, 11, 12, and 13.

The above observations lead us to the conclusion that shoes which are not adapted to the foot of each individual are defective ; and that a shoemaker who would excel in his art, and who desires to furnish his customers with a perfect article, ought to have an exact knowledge of every diversity of form, more especially if he wishes to prevent corns upon the joints and between the toes, inflammation of the roots of the nails (onychia), especially of the great toes, and painful callosities. He will prevent all these annoyances by giving a proper form to his shoes : the toes will not then be bent, the nails will not be compressed, the joint of the great toe and the foot itself will no longer be subject to tumours and swellings, and the skin of the foot generally will be preserved from abrasion. I say further, if the shoemaker be intelligent, if he thoroughly understand his business, or have a clear conception of progression; if he can distinguish the natural from a faulty form of the foot, he will be enabled to correct any defect in his work, and preserve his customers from much torture, as well as save them from falls, bruises, and sprains. The evil results produced by ill-formed shoes, as now enumerated, must convince us of the importance of a radical reform in the manner in which they are at present made, and of the propriety of obtaining them of the best possible fashion.

My readers may, nevertheless, be surprised at finding a professor of medicine condescending to treat so humble a subject; but I flatter myself that their astonishment will cease if they peruse these pages; when they will be made aware of the immense amount of knowledge necessary to deal worthily with so important a subject. I would have them remember that the great Xenophon has not disdained to transmit to posterity judicious instructions as to the best manner of preserving the feet of the horse. A Duke of Newcastle, and other distinguished persons, have prided themselves upon their knowledge of the hoof of this animal, and have bestowed much study upon the iron shoe necessary. Our feet are certainly of as much value as those of that noble animal ; and a proper charity begins at home. It is, then, to mankind that I devote my attention and care. I labour for the benefit of my fellow-creatures ; and this motive, united with the example of the two great names I have cited above, gives dignity to my work, and justifies my exertions. I propose, in the first place, to consider scientifically, the foot, and our mode of progression ; then to treat of shoes and boots, as worn by men, women, and children, and to enlarge upon their most proper form. The diseases and discomfort occasioned by ill-made shoes, with the means of prevention and cure, will occupy the concluding portion of this little treatise.

NOTE.—This little memoir may be considered as a supplement to my "Dissertation upon the Physical Education of Children," published in Vol. vii. of the "Memoirs of the Academy of Haarlem."

# THE FOOT.

## CHAPTER I.

It is not necessary to give here a minute anatomical description of the foot, which our readers may study for themselves in the magnificent works of Albinus, Cheselden, or Sue; but a brief account is indispensable to the clear understanding of the subsequent observations.

The foot (Fig. 1) is divided into three parts, of which the principal, $N$, $E$, is called the Tarsus; $E$, $D$, the Metatarsus; and $D$, $A$, the Toes. The tarsus is composed of seven bones; the metatarsus contains five; and each of the toes consists of three small bones, except the great toe, which has but two. Beneath the articulation of the great toe, with the metatarsus, $D$, there are two small bones, $K$, which are called the Lenticular, or Sesamoïd bones, because of their resemblance to the seed of the plant Sesame, whence the ancient Greeks derived the name.

The seven bones of the tarsus are capable of very little movement; those of the metatarsus have much more; and the bones of the toes are as mobile as those of the fingers. I remember seeing at Amsterdam, twenty-five years ago, a man who had, in place of arms, merely short immovable appendages, and who executed with his feet all those actions for which we employ our fingers. He could write, cut his own pens, fire a pistol, &c. The late Professor Roëll dissected these rudimentary arms, and made a demonstration of their anatomical deficiencies in my presence. Ulysses Aldrovandus has given several instances of this kind, in his "History of Deformities," in chapter iv., *upon deformities of the arms and hands:* the cases there mentioned, of a woman who used her toes in place of her fingers, and of a certain Thomas Schnueiter, are very remarkable.

The arrangement of the bones and muscles of the feet prove that we might make use of them in many ways, were those members not so entirely neglected, and rendered useless by shoes and boots, constructed, as it were, on purpose to destroy their mechanism.

The ancient Greeks seem to have injured their feet by sandals, κρηπιδα, or *solea*, as well as by shoes, ὑποδηγατα, or *calceus*, as appears from the works of Celsus, Paulus Ægineta, and others.

The great toe is naturally shorter than the second toe, but not to the extent sometimes represented in ancient statues and the drawings of artists of the sixteenth century, who have, in sketching the foot, drawn it as of a lozenge form, much pointed in front.

The shoes of both sexes are made upon the same principle — more or less pointed, according to the fashion of the time, but always in such a manner that the four smaller toes are closely pressed together and against the great toe, so that they frequently ride one over the other, for want of space.

Not only the toes, but the five bones of the metatarsus, or instep, lose, from this cause, their form and mobility. The seven bones of the tarsus suffer less, but they are injured by the use of high heels, especially among women, as I shall prove in the succeeding chapters.

If we consider the sole of the foot (Fig. 8), we shall see that the diagonal line of this supposed lozenge does not pass through its centre, but that the exterior portion, $A$, $B$, $D$, $M$, Fig. 8, considerably exceeds the interior, $A$, $B$, $E$, $N$.

The Last on which the shoe is made having to serve for both feet, is, nevertheless, always shaped in such a manner that the two sides are nearly alike, so that the great toe, strong as it is, is forced towards the others, and sensibly turned in, which renders it much less useful in walking. This causes the large tumours, or bunions, that rise at $D$ (Fig. 1), or at $E$, Fig. 8, from which we suffer cruelly when our shoes are too narrow, inflammations frequently resulting, which prevent our walking for some time. Fashion inflicts these agonies upon its votaries, and vanity stifles the expression of their sufferings.

The sole of the foot is naturally so formed that on the inside we rest only upon the heel and the articulation of the bones of the instep with the toes, and externally upon the tuberosity of the bone of the metatarsus, where it joins the little toe at $A$.

All these parts touch the ground upon the line $A$, $B$, (Fig. 1). This line lengthens in walking; and it is the neglect of this lengthening by shoemakers that causes all the pain and disfigurement of our feet.

In those who wear high heels, this line, $A$, $B$, is made to assume a concave form, as at $B$, $V$, $T$, $U$ (Fig. 3), which occasions a multiplicity of evils, of which I will speak after I have fully described the structure of the foot.

## CHAPTER II.

### BONES OF THE FOOT.

IF we examine the arrangement of the bones of the foot (Fig. 1), we see at a glance that the bone of the heel, $N$, $M$, $I$, touches the ground, as do also the lenticular bone, $K$, and the great toe, $A$, $C$, and that all these points fall upon the line $A$, $B$. The astragalus, $R$, $M$, $I$, which supports at $R$ the whole weight of the body, is thus sustained by two oblique lines, $R$, $B$, $R$, $A$ (Fig. 3), when there results, when we stand erect, or still more if we lift a weight, a slight depression of the point $R$ towards the ground, and the two points $A$ and $B$ recede slightly from each other. The line $A$, $B$, is thus lengthened, so that, did the hollow of the foot touch the ground, the lines $R$, $B$, and $R$, $C$, united, would equal $B$, $N$. It is, therefore, evident that a shoe which is an exact fit when we are seated, will pinch the foot cruelly between $N$, $B$, and $A$, $O$ (Fig. 1), as soon as we attempt to stand in it, especially if the quarter does not yield backwards, which is partly opposed by the tie or buckle; although, in general, the heel does recede, when the shoe gets misshapen and trodden down.

The change which takes place in the foot when we walk is of great importance: the great toe, $A$, $K$

(Fig. 2), then rests upon the ground; the metatarsus, or instep, rises from $b$ to $B$; and the line $d$, $c$, lengthens and extends to $B$, increasing the interval $c$, $B$, which is in this figure $\frac{1}{4}$ of an inch French measure, and, in consequence, a whole inch in nature.

The three first and the sixth of the figures in my Plate are taken from the work of the great Albinus, upon the Skeleton and Muscles, and are one-quarter the natural size.

The soles of our shoes and boots, which are generally made of the strongest leather, become, in consequence of this elongation of the foot, too short in proportion. The shoe then pinches the heel, and produces still worse effects upon all the toes, especially the great toe; for as the sole cannot yield from $c$ to $B$, $A$ yields towards $c$, and the great toe is bent as at $f$, forming the angle $e$, $f$, $D$, together with the rest of the toes. Thus are produced corns upon the joints, and other painful deformities of the feet.

The faster we walk, the more will the sole be shortened, inasmuch as $C$, $B$, always continue proportioned to one another.

It follows, therefore, that every boot and shoe ought to be $\frac{1}{2}$ an inch or an inch longer than $A$, $B$, which is the exact length of the foot as the shoemaker measures it in repose. From habit or custom he usually adds a few lines; but this addition depends upon a mere guess, which is not founded upon any principle, as he is ignorant of the true elongation of the foot as I have proved it to exist.

This elongation, indeed, is not the same in all persons, and it is consequently most necessary to take the measure of $A$, $b$, first, with the rule, and then with a strip of leather or cloth, from $A$, $b$, to $B$, when the foot is bent, as in Fig. 2, from $b$, $B$, to determine the length of sole necessary. The addition usually made by shoemakers is only $\frac{1}{24}$ of the whole length of the foot, whereas it should be at least $\frac{1}{12}$.

If we examine the feet of persons shod according to the present fashion of high heels, we shall perceive that they do not rest upon the ground in the line $A$, $B$ (Fig. 3), but that they describe the curved line $B$, $V$, $T$, $a$, because of the height of the heel, $V$, $S$; and as the weight of the whole body rests upon $V$, $S$, the instep suffers in consequence. The foot is thus no longer of the natural length, $B$, $A$, but of $d$, $a$, $b$, having lost the length of the line $W$, $a$; that is to say, $\frac{2}{3}$ of the height of the heel, $V$, $S$. The instep is thus made more convex, more rounded, which is esteemed a peculiar beauty, and the foot not only appears, but is actually rendered smaller.

Curvature of the foot to this extent cannot be effected without submitting the bones composing it to considerable changes, influencing chiefly those of the tarsus, especially the heel-bone and the head of the astragalus, $H$ and $L$.

It is more than probable that in those persons whose feet have not been distorted by the use of high heels, the heel-bone receives the anterior part of the astragalus ($H$, Fig. 1) upon the eminence $M$, $L$, which is then divided into two small sinuses ($E$ and $F$, Fig. 4), separated by a space, $K$. Very frequently, however, we find but one sinus, as at $E$, $F$, Fig. 5. We naturally inquire which of these formations is the natural one.

The celebrated Vesalius has distinctly represented and described these two sinuses or depressions.

Albinus mentions them particularly in his smaller work upon the Bones, but in the illustrations to his work on the Skeleton, he has represented one only. Winslow mentions but one; and Sue, in his engravings illustrative of the works of Monro, gives one only. Bidloo shows two in his drawing of the heel-bone, Pl. 105 of his work on Anatomy.

It appears to me very probable, then, that these sinuses become united from the pressure to which they are subjected by high heels, causing the obliteration of the division $K$.

I possess the heel-bones of a new-born infant and of a child of two years of age, in both of which the two sinuses are distinctly marked. Albinus has represented them double, in his drawings of the bones of children. It is therefore evident that they are frequently, and probably more often, double than single, though I have always found them united in the feet of those accustomed to wear high heels.

In the skeleton of a lame man in my possession, the sinuses are united in the heel-bone of the lame leg. In that of the right, which was the healthy side, they are distinct. The reason of this is, that in this man the lame leg was, as in the case of persons wearing high heels, supported solely by the toes.

The head of the astragalus ($H$, Fig. 3) in the feet of those who wear heels, is bent downwards, and this happens most easily to young persons, in whose feet the neck of the astragalus is still entirely cartilaginous. The navicular and cuneiform bones are also affected; and the worst result of this is, that the surfaces of these bones, and of those of the metatarsus which are in contact with them, are considerably diminished, and so distorted from their natural position, that they can never be restored to it. This is the reason why those who have been long accustomed to wear high heels suffer great pain in the calf of the leg, when compelled to move barefooted or in low-heeled shoes, the muscles of this part, *gastrocnemius cum soleo*, which form the tendon Achilles, being incapable of enduring the unaccustomed stretching.

All that we have stated is as applicable to women as to men: in them the great toe becomes bent towards $p$, precisely as in men; and the higher the heels, the greater will be the distortion,—the centre of gravity, $R$, acting more and more in the line $R$, $a$; and the higher the heel and the smaller the sole, the greater becomes the risk of falls and sprains. Of this truth we have daily experience; and it will be found that all pedestrians and persons obliged to be much in motion prefer low-heeled shoes.

The celebrated André, in his excellent "Traité d'Orthopédie," remarks that high heels are very apt to induce curvature of the spine in young girls, who ought never to be allowed to wear them before the age of fifteen. He adds, that tight shoes or boots ought to be considered as highly prejudicial to the figure, as in consequence of, and to avoid the pain and inconvenience they cause, young girls will frequently twist their bodies into constrained and unnatural attitudes. Similar results are produced in men who wear heels of an extravagant height.

As the leg rests on the foot, and the centre of gravity acts in a line perpendicularly, a line designated by Borelli *linea propensionis*, and represented by $R$, $S$, in Figs. 3 and 6, it follows that this line ought always to be observed. The heels, $B$, $T$, $b$, Fig. 6, must be advanced under the foot beyond the line $R$, $S$, and in length ought to be at least a quarter of that of the foot.

When the heels are made smaller, *i.e.*, when they do not reach to $R$, $S$, but only as far as $V$, $Y$, they

## BONES OF THE FOOT.

do not support the centre of gravity,—the sole of the shoe is then subjected to considerable strain, and the heel receding, soon becomes detached from the sole at *T, V*.

Formerly, when women wore high wooden heels, much sloped both in front and behind, so as to finish in a narrow point, *S*, Fig. 3, it was found that if the heel was placed too far forward, as at *Z*, the foot fell back; if it were placed too far back, as at *b*, it caused insupportable pain in the toes. This is an additional proof that the heel ought always to be so placed as to support the centre of gravity represented by the line *R, S*, Fig. 3.

High heels have a further most serious inconvenience for females approaching the term of their pregnancy. To maintain the erect position, females in this interesting situation are compelled to carry the head and shoulders backwards, when the spinal column becomes relatively more curved and hollow inferiorly, and the pelvis or haunches more straight, inasmuch as the lumbar vertebræ, where they are connected with the os sacrum, which forms the posterior part of the pelvis, are pushed forward into or over this cavity. The head of the child, which has to pass through the strait of the pelvis, is then more or less impeded at the best, and is often so thoroughly wedged and obstructed there, that it has to be brought down with instruments, which, however well contrived, must always accomplish the end of their application with force, that may readily prove hurtful to the mother or the child, if not perchance to both.

I am intimately persuaded that the custom of wearing high heels, solely intended to give height to the figure, especially of the fair sex, is the cause of many difficult labours, more particularly among the wealthy. Women in the lower ranks of life do not suffer in the same way, escaping mainly, as I apprehend, from the habit of wearing low-heeled boots and shoes.

The centre of gravity of the whole body is displaced by unreasonably high heels. It no longer coincides with the centre of movement, but is raised in proportion to the height of the heels. Persons so shod must, therefore, walk less securely; they are more apt to fall and sprain the ankle; and thus, I believe, are caused many cases of fracture of the patella, or knee-cap, which, common enough among women at Amsterdam, happens very rarely to men; unless, indeed, it be among the porters, who mount the stairs of the warehouses, charged with heavy burthens. The curious may find a full account of many accidents caused by thus disturbing the centre of gravity of the body in my "Mémoire sur l'Education Physique des Enfans," printed in the "Mem. de l'Acad. de Haarlem," tom. vii.; and all that concerns fracture of the patella in my Latin dissertation "De Patella fracta," published in 1754.

PLATE II.

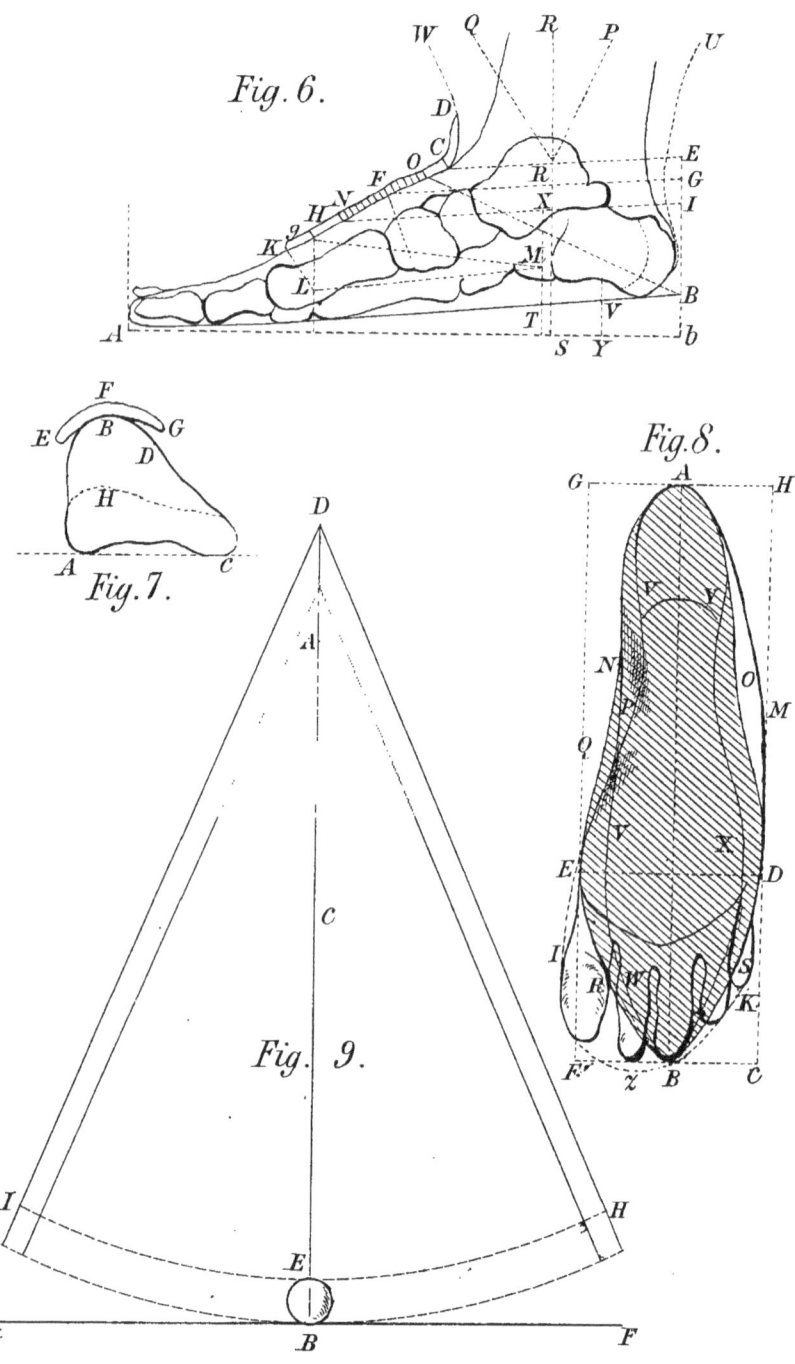

## CHAPTER III.

#### OF THE SOLE OF THE FOOT.

The sole of the foot is generally of the form represented in Fig. 8; the part comprising the toes, $E$, $D$, $B$, in $F$, $E$, occupying about one-third of the whole length of the foot; although on this matter painters are not generally agreed among themselves. Occasionally they even neglect their own rules; for Albert Durer, who adopts the proportion of a third in his first book " On the Proportions of the Human Figure," page 55, makes it two-sevenths on page 22.

Jean de Wit, who painted so exquisitely in grisaille, has published a very worthless book on the Human Proportions, which the Dutch follow for want of a better guide; and, indeed, there is nothing satisfactory since the time of Durer. In the profile of the man, Pl. III., De Wit has given more than a third of the foot to the toes; but in that of the woman, which is a bad copy of the Venus de Medicis, he has given an accurate third, as Durer has done. In the drawing of the Venus in vol. iii. of the "Pl. du Dictionnaire Encyclopédique," Pl. 39, Fig. 9, we find two-sevenths for the toes. In the figure of the Antinous, again, Pl. 34, Figs. 9 and 10, the proportion is one-third. In the Farnese Hercules the toes are still larger. In my own foot they are about one-third.

The toes are naturally all parallel to the diameter $A$, $B$, as I have represented them in Fig. 8, which is the outline of a foot that has not been distorted by ill-made shoes. Albert Durer, however, who seems only to have seen feet deformed by ill-treatment, gives the toes an oblique direction (*Ib.* p. 55); as if nature were bound to follow our absurd caprices.

In all feet the second toe, or one next the great toe, is longer than the others, and also a little raised above them; but a short shoe forces this toe back, and at the same time causes it to take an oblique direction; and this is the reason why not only Albert Durer and De Wit, but the great Albinus, have represented it as deformed and thrust inwards. They have fallen into this error, because they have neglected the study of the antique. We may instance the Farnese Hercules, the Antinous, the Gladiator, and the Venus de Medicis, as copies of undistorted and natural beauty. Vesalius, Genga, and Sue, have followed nature correctly. There is no doubt that the second toe, $Z$, Fig. 8, ought always to be longer than the great toe, $F$. The ancients, whose feet were not so distorted by the simple sole or sandal, always represent it thus in all their statues, as do also those modern artists who have

## THE SOLE OF THE FOOT. 23

been most attentive to natural beauty. I may instance the exquisite wood engravings of Vesalius, and the etchings of Genga and Sue.

The Dutch peasantry are in the habit of making a differently-shaped shoe for each foot, that is to say, they always make the sole right and left. They cut it of the form, *A*, *M*, *D*, *K*, *B*, *I*, *E*, *Q*, *N*, *A*, Fig. 8, which is most sensible, as it agrees exactly with the natural form of our feet. Sabots, which were probably the first shoes invented, are always made upon the same principles.

There is an old and most unreasonable custom of making the shoes for both feet alike, from one and the same last, with the additional absurdity of giving the sole a certain arbitrary form, as at *A*, *O*, *D*, *S*, *B*, *R*, *E*, *N*, Fig. 8. This produces the most deplorable consequences: the great toe is pushed violently in the direction *E*, *R*, *B*, and the little toe towards *D*, *S*, *B*; the other toes are forced to encroach one upon the other, and exchange their cylindrical for a quadrangular form. Secondly, the foot is pushed beyond the sole, *A*, *O*, *D*, as far as *A*, *M*, *D*, and the joint of the great toe swells, and is distorted from its natural position at *E*. Another disadvantage is, the uneven way in which young persons thus shod wear their shoes: the heel treads over the sole, either to the inside or the outside, because the diagonal of the motion of the foot no longer coincides with that of the shoe; and all these particulars are immensely increased when high heels are worn.

I think I have thus proved that shoes made upon the same last for both feet must cause distortion; that changing the shoes from one foot to the other cannot remedy the defects of the soles; and that we thus cripple ourselves, and render our feet useless for many other purposes besides easy walking. Their formation, which is but a modification of that of the hands, clearly proves this. J. Ketel, one of our most celebrated portrait-painters, painted first with his hands and afterwards with his feet and toes. And in North Holland, I have heard of a girl born without arms, who did all kinds of work with her toes.*

* Miss Biffin, a celebrated miniature-painter of London, who died at Liverpool, October, 1850, executed all her works with her toes, being destitute of arms. The Chinese and Hindoos will pick up the smallest objects, such as pins and needles, with their toes, if their hands happen to be occupied.—*Translator*.

## CHAPTER IV.

### OF WALKING IN GENERAL.

The erect position being a necessary prelude to walking progression, it may be well, in discussing this subject, to look to what the celebrated Borelli has left us in his excellent work on the Animal Motions.*

Our principal business being to explain the manner in which we raise our feet from the ground in walking, we may turn to Fig. 9, where $A$, $C$, $B$ represents the length of the leg and foot, turning upon the hip-joint at $A$. $C$ indicates the knee. Let us imagine that a man standing on his right foot begins to walk along the street, $G$, $F$, it is certain that if there should be a stone, $E$, $B$, at $B$, he will strike his foot against it; but if the heel of the shoe should be of the height $E$, $B$, the centre of movement at the hip being thus raised to $D$, he will avoid it, because the foot will pass from $H$ to $I$. It may therefore be concluded that high heels may be of some service to those who have to walk much on stony ground, or who live in cities, the streets of which are unevenly paved; inasmuch as where the whole sole is flat and without

---

* Borelli "De Motu Animalium." 4to. Rom., 1680.

heel, the points of the toes will be more apt to come in contact with the inequalities. This was probably the reason why, in the olden times, shoes were made with the points turned up,—a fashion which still prevails, indeed, where sabots or wooden shoes are worn.

It seems clear that we are more liable to knock our toes against the stones as we move more quickly; whence it follows that one who only walks leisurely in his garden, and is borne from house to house seated in a carriage, may wear the kind of shoe he likes; but the pedestrian from necessity, need not imitate the great in this.

Thick cork soles have been proposed, but have never been much in vogue; for they are extremely incommodious in walking, by reason of their thickness; and then cork does not keep out the wet, and snow penetrates and fills its pores, so that in winter it is especially objectionable.

Returning to the former fashion of turning up the point of the shoe, I may be permitted to refer to the custom which still obtains in the South of France of turning up the tips of the shoes of mules, with a view to keeping them clear of the loose stones and asperities of the road, and to our own practice of bending up the front of our skate-irons, that we may not butt against and be caught by every little roughness and inequality of the ice.

These considerations being inferences from the physics of progressive motion, may be taken as general rules, and are of course only applicable where foot-gear of the kind described is worn.

The wealthy walk (as we have shown in Fig. 3), by reason of the height of their heels, on the fore-ends of their feet only; and, consequently, very badly; they walk, if I may be allowed the comparison, in the same way as the greater number of the lower animals—on their toes only. The high heel may keep the toes from inequalities and rolling stones, but he who wears it can never walk at his ease, save, perhaps, on a carpeted floor or the smoothest pavement; enough to demonstrate the advantages of broad and low heels, which are in universal use by those who have to walk much and long. It is only the lame, indeed, affected in a particular way, who require a high heel, in aid of a natural defect. With them there is a physical necessity for walking on the toes; and then the high heel becomes a support and a comfort. I am even of opinion that it is advisable, under such circumstances, to have recourse to a raised heel in early life; for, without it, the knee of the healthy limb is preternaturally bent in walking, which is not only unsightly, but further adds force to the descent of the crippled limb every time it is brought to the ground, and causes the head of the thigh to be pushed higher than is proper, and the foot to shrink. Nor in some cases is it merely necessary to place the support under the proper heel-bone, but to bring it forward under the toes, *a*, *U*, Fig. 3, as *a*, *U*, *r*, *q*; for the more evenly the two feet are raised from the ground, provided the body be strong enough, the more natural and easy is the act of walking.

NOTE.—In speaking of foot-gear it seems very proper not only to think of those whom nature has sent into the world perfect in their lower extremities, but of those also to whom she has been less kind, and furnished with feet more or less deformed. Professor Camper, accordingly, here gives a chapter on clubfoot, the cause of which he finds in a want of sufficient space within the mother's womb; whereby the bones of the feet, and especially the neck of the astragalus, are so displaced and distorted, that experience has assured him of the difficulty of restoring them to their natural shape and position, and anatomy has even demonstrated the impossibility, in certain cases, of doing so. In dissecting the body of a child affected with clubfoot, in 1777, he says: "I found that the two astragaluses had undergone a great degree of compression in their necks, *H*, Fig. 1, whereby the forepart of the foot was strongly drawn inwards by the tibialis anticus and tibialis posticus muscles, which unite over the wedge-shaped bone, *E*, *G*, at *F*, and over the tuberosity of the navicular bone, *G*, Fig. 1. The fibular or outside muscles thereby lose much of their force, and are made incapable of drawing the foot outwards, in consequence of which the astragalus is pushed still more inwards, and further crippled. But this is not all: the calcaneum, or heel-bone, becomes even oblique in its position, and its tuberosity, *N*, Fig. 1, is curved towards *B*, by the short flexor and adductor of the great toe. The length of the lever, *I*, *N*, is thereby evidently shortened, and the tendon Achilles at the same time loses power. In these facts lie the true reasons of the difficulty of overcoming and curing this vicious conformation. The contraction of the foot, and of the heel especially, is such that many club-footed persons can by no means touch the ground with the heel; the muscles, naturally antagonistic and balancing each other, having their equality of power destroyed. M. Vander Haar, of Bois le Duc, has contrived a variety of machines in wood for the cure of club-feet, and in cases of little severity they seem to answer. Cheselden has proposed a very commodious bandage; and others have described steel boots and various machines, all of which may have their merits in particular cases; but I am obliged to confess, in favour of truth, that with all or any of these, I have only succeeded very rarely in doing good. The steel boxes, which I have tried in especial, I have found useless;—patients too often continue to go about, not on the sole, but on the outer edge of the foot,—the sole, instead of being applied to the ground, being even turned upwards. The feet and legs of club-footed persons are always smaller and more slender than proper; for what reason I know not, for there is no apparent defect in the nutrition of the parts, neither is there any compression of the nerves, that might arrest the flow of the hypothetical nervous juice or animal spirit."

So far our Professor on this subject, so important to those who suffer and to those who are intrusted with finding a remedy. Modern science has happily done much since Camper lived and wrote. *Tenotomy*, or subcutaneous section of the tendons of the rebellious muscles, whereby we now work such marvellous cures, was not thought of in his day. The curious on this subject will find it exhausted in the works of Dr. Little on Club-foot and other deformities.—*Translator*.

## CHAPTER V.

### OF THE BOOT AND SHOE.

Boots and shoes are divided into the soles, to which are attached the heels and upper leathers. The upper leather is divided into the *vamp*, or front, and the *quarter*, or hind-part, with which are connected the ears, whereby the shoe is fastened over the instep on to the foot. *Vide* Fig. 6, $A$, $X$, $T$, $A$, &c.; $C$, $D$, &c.

With regard to the *quarter*, we may observe, that when the fastening is made as high as possible, as at $F$, $C$, the upper edge, $C$, $E$, is parallel to $A$, $B$, and the lower part, $F$, $H$, $M$, $T$, is sewed to the vamp, so that $H$ is parallel to $C$, $E$. The direction in which the sole of the shoe then comes to be fastened to the foot, is in the line $O$, $B$; when the shoe embraces the great part of the foot, and the tendon Achilles, or posterior aspect of the heel, is not painfully compressed at $E$. With such a shoe, he who has not much walking, and little running up and down stairs, may get on well enough; but the foot will look extremely long.

When the fastening is situated at $K$, $H$, the line in which it acts will be that of $g$, $B$, and the upper edge of the quarter will be, *H, I*, at so small a distance from the bottom of the shoe, that it must be impossible to secure it firmly to the foot; it must either severely pinch the heel at *J*, or it will be so loose that the heel will jerk out at every step. This position of the fastening, therefore, is the least proper; notwithstanding which, it is that which is preferred by all classes, particularly by sailors and persons of rank of both sexes.

In the third position, the buckle or fastening will be placed midway between each of those that have been described, viz., at *O, N*, and will be over the middle of the instep, whereby it will never be felt as an inconvenience; 1st, because the shoe will keep well on; 2nd, because in the motions of the foot backwards towards *R, P*, or forwards towards *R, Q*, there will be less constraint about *G*, by reason of the small amount of movement which the tendon Achilles suffers in such circumstances. On the other hand, when the fastening is made so high as *C, F*, the upper edge of the quarter will cause much inconvenience when the foot is forcibly stretched out. 3rd, The buckle or fastening will then prove a source of no inconvenience when the leg is bent forward, as in mounting a stair or a slope, inasmuch as it will be below the crease which the leg forms with the foot, and will not press upon the tendons of the anterior muscles of the leg which move the foot and extend the toes. The best position for the buckle or fastening of a shoe is, therefore, directly over the top of the instep, neither too high nor too low, exactly over the spot where the triangular ligament connects the tendons of the extensors of the toes with the bones of the tarsus and metatarsus, at $O$, $N$, a spot which Albinus indicates by $\kappa$, $\lambda$, in the 9th plate of his great work on the muscles. A shoe made and secured in this way will certainly cause the smallest amount of inconvenience possible, whether it be in running or walking, in ascending or in descending, and will therefore be preferable to one made and fastened in any other way.

All that has now been said applies indifferently to the shoes of men and women; though convenience and propriety do not always carry it against appearance and fashion. The shoes of women would undoubtedly be best fastened over the middle of the instep, as in men; but the foot would then be held to appear too large or clumsy; and so the shoe, when worn with a buckle or fastening, has it over the roots of the toes, the quarter of the shoe being very long, and the heel tending to escape with every step.

The shoes of children ought to be made, from the first, in such a manner as to support the foot without compressing it anywhere. All those parts which finally assume a bony structure are, in infancy, not only cartilaginous, but of the most delicate texture. Our feet are often distorted by ill-made shoes before we are a year old. Savages, and those who let their children go barefoot, preserve them from these evils.

Locke does not mention the form of shoes proper for children; he merely wishes them to be made very thin.* He criticises, in his excellent "Treatise upon the Education of Children," the feet of the Chinese women, ascribing to them their bad health and frequent falls. Nevertheless, it is a fact that we give to our children, even before they are a year old, shoes made upon the same last for both feet, which must of necessity not only hurt, but destroy the tender and delicate bones of their feet, especially those of the toes; and as they grow older, we continue to give them shoes still more calculated, from the stiffness of the upper-leathers and unpliable nature of the soles, to confirm this bending of the toes and deformity of the whole foot.

I was astonished, on reading the "Prize Treatise" of M. Balaxerd, to see that he recommends that from the age of three to ten years, children should wear sabots, without heels; attributing the crookedness of the feet of most children to the pernicious practice of wearing high heels.

It is true that sabots are always made of a distinct shape for each foot; but is it probable that a foot,

---

* Locke's reason for this—*i. e.*, "that they may thus be more easily wetted"—will have no credit in the present age. We are now far enough advanced in knowledge to appreciate the great advantage of dry and warm feet.—*Translator.*

still of a delicate and for the most part cartilaginous texture, should develop itself advantageously in a heavy mass of wood, utterly destitute of flexibility?

Of late years, persons of the upper classes have adopted the custom of letting their children go barefoot, at least in the house, a practice which I much commend.

NOTE.—When I wrote upon the Physical Education of Children, I mentioned only casually their shoes; I had not then turned my attention to the subject, otherwise I should have dwelt more at length upon the best form of shoes for these delicate beings; as I am now convinced that the injury to our feet commences from the moment we begin to walk.—*Author.*

## CHAPTER VI.

#### OF THE BEST SHAPE OF A SHOE.

The result of the observations detailed in the preceding chapters is, to prove to us that shoes fitted for the use of those engaged in active pursuits must possess, firstly, a sole properly proportioned to the length necessary to allow of the elongation of the foot when in motion—from $c$ to $B$, Fig. 2; the shoemaker first taking the measure of the foot in repose, and then that of the same foot when bent, as we have shown it in Fig. 2.

Secondly. A different last must be used for each foot.

Thirdly. The true dimensions of the foot ($E$, $D$, $N$, $M$, Fig. 8) ought to be taken with callipers, or bent compasses. In this we should be following the example of the best wigmakers of Paris, who use these means to ensure an accurate fit.

Most shoemakers err in making the soles too narrow. They trust to the stretching of the upper-leathers, thinking that they thus produce a closer fit, and avoid creases, troubling themselves very little about the suffering they thus occasion. The sole, $A$, $N$, $E$, $R$, $B$, $S$, $D$, $O$, Fig. 8, which I have copied from the latest Parisian pattern, intended for the sole of the foot, $A, I, Z, K, M, A$, Fig. 8, will prove my assertion.

Fourthly. The sole ought always to be as broad as is possible, consistently with a becoming appearance.

Fifthly. The point of the sole ought to be a little raised, so as to aid in avoiding inequality of ground.

Sixthly. The heel ought to be of a moderate height, and placed well forward, so as to support the centre of gravity.

Seventhly. The vamp and quarters ought to be so proportioned, that the buckle or fastening lies over the wedge-shaped bone, exactly at the spot where this bone and the bones of the metatarsus of the great toe and the two others next it are united; that is to say, at $E$, Fig. 1.

Shoes made in this manner will enable the wearer to walk with ease and safety, and would prevent corns, bunions, and strained insteps, as well as many sprains, and injuries to the tendons of the extensor muscles of the toes.

I cannot improve upon the description given above, of the advantages to be gained from shoes made after this model.

We are all obliged, in some measure, to obey the dictates of custom and fashion; but if we wish to flatter our vanity, by appearing taller than we are by nature, or if we desire to render our feet smaller than they ought to be according to the just proportions of our figure, or if we insist upon giving to our feet a form contrary to all the uses for which they are destined, we must resign ourselves to the discomforts and painful diseases occasioned by improperly-shaped shoes; which cannot be avoided by means short of a miracle.

It is absolutely necessary that the soles of children's shoes should be made very broad, and round, rather than pointed in front. All stiffness and harshness of the upper-leathers are also extremely pernicious.

The upper-leathers should always be made of a yielding material; and if, for the sake of durability, we choose a strong leather, we ought to take care that the shoemaker does not stretch it too tightly upon the last, and especially forbid him to wet it: as the leather dries it will shrink, and cruelly pinch the foot. By these precautions we may counterbalance, in some measure, defects in the shape of the sole; and if we insist upon voluntarily submitting ourselves to an absurd and painful slavery, we may yet, in some degree, alleviate our sufferings.

I have thought it well to be thus particular, because the remedies which surgery supplies are of little use; it is far better to be beforehand with the mischief, and rather to prevent or diminish its causes.

## CHAPTER VII.

### OF THE INCONVENIENCES OCCASIONED BY ILL-MADE SHOES, AND THEIR REMEDIES.

THE Author of Nature has protected the soles of our feet, even before we are born, by bestowing upon them a thicker skin, and a cuticle or outer skin, stronger than that of the rest of the body. This outer skin becomes sensibly thicker in those who go barefoot; and, by a curious provision, instead of wearing away, as is the case in other inanimate substances, if they are exposed to friction, it becomes more and more thick and callous.

Shoes and boots, however well made, will chafe and press upon the foot, especially upon those parts which, from the thinness of the cuticle, are not calculated to endure much friction; and thus are occasioned corns and bunions. A bunion is endurable so long as it is not inflamed; but when that happens, it is intolerable.

Should a callosity of this description form upon the heel, from the pressure of the edge of the shoe, the sole being too narrow, we must, in the first place, procure a proper shoe, and seek to remove the malady by emollient remedies,—by a soap plaster and the like; but if we do not begin by removing the pressure of the sole, we shall hope in vain for a cure.

One of my friends, residing in Amsterdam, suffered from a bunion, all attempts to cure which were in vain tried for more than a year. The sufferer was forced to keep the house, and neglect his business, in consequence of the insupportable pain he suffered in walking. When I was summoned, I examined the foot, and the callous mass which had formed upon the anterior portion of the great toe. I made a species of receptacle of cork for the diseased toe, carefully removing with a file every particle which could press upon it. This little contrivance was fastened to the toe, so as to protect it entirely from injury, and proved entirely successful. My patient found himself immediately able to attend to his affairs, without pain or inconvenience; and in six months, a complete cure was effected; the emollient remedies producing their good effect from the moment that all pressure was removed.

A similar cure of a case in which the external surface, $D$, $K$, Fig. 8, was affected, confirmed the excellence of this method of procedure.

It sometimes happens that, when the part $H$, $I$, or $F$, $G$, Fig. 6, is much compressed by the fastening of the shoe or the seam, $E$, $B$, the heel over the tendon Achilles, although already protected by a callosity, becomes tender and inflamed. In such a case, an embrocation of oil and white wine or vinegar may be applied, in order to soften and remove the swelling ; but, above all, the cause of the evil must be removed, by wearing shoes or boots which do not press upon the part.

The torture inflicted upon the large joint of the great toe, when the sole is too short and the upper-leather is hard and unyielding, is infinitely more cruel. The joint becomes red and swollen ; and I have frequently observed that the little synovial sac, or bursa, which naturally exists at this spot, as also under the elbow and over the kneecap, becomes filled with a fluid. The same thing will sometimes happen to the articulation of the little toe with the bone of the foot. A large shoe is here of the first necessity, and an embrocation or liniment similar to that prescribed for the heel may be used with benefit.

When the sole is too short and the upper-leather stiff, so that the shoe or boot will yield neither at the toe nor heel, inflammation of the root of the great toe-nail is occasioned, which is intensely painful, and callosities grow under and around the nail. I have seen some in which the nail was buried to the depth of a quarter of an inch. The nail must be carefully cut away from the callosity. The inflammation will disappear of itself, as soon as the pressure is removed, as will also the callosities ; but they may be softened by the use of the soap plaster. It is dangerous to touch these callosities with caustic

# EFFECTS OF ILL-MADE SHOES.

or butter of antimony, as they will then frequently become malignant and difficult to cure.

The disease is not caused by any primary degeneration, but is a consequence of perpetual pressure: the toe is, as it were, forced to incur the disease; and it is above all necessary here to remove the cause, in order to prevent its effects.

The commonest and most painful affection of the feet are corns, which have been well described by C. Celsus, P. Ægineta, and Ætius. They appear most frequently upon the prominent joints of the toes, as at $f$ and $p$, in Figs. 2 and 3, and upon the side of the little toe, $s$, Fig. 8. The epidermis is naturally very thin upon these parts, but by constant pressure it becomes thickened and horny. The progress of this affection is as follows:—At first the hardened portion is of the size of a pin's head; a second thickening ensues, and it continues thus until a species of thorn is formed, which compresses the tendinous expansion of the covering of the joint, causing horrible pain—with which my readers are probably better acquainted by experience than they could become by the most minute description I might give. Corns also grow between the toes, where they touch each other; and they sometimes attack the sole of the foot. Wherever placed, they render walking extremely painful.

Well-made and easy shoes are, in all these cases, the best remedy; and in addition, the application of some soap plaster spread upon soft thick leather, will be found very useful.*

It may seem superfluous to observe that the indurated skin should be previously removed with a penknife, as this will considerably hasten the cure.

Celsus recommends (book v., chap. 28), that corns shall be first scraped with a knife, and then anointed with resin. Paulus Ægineta has devoted a whole chapter to the subject (book iv., chap. 80). He agrees with Celsus, but proposes pumice-stone, instead of the knife, to remove the surface of the corn; and then the application of various emollient and astringent remedies, as the *atramentum hitorium*, which much resembled our common ink, and contained vitriol. He also advises the use of cantharides. The fame of these insects for the cure of warts and such fungous excrescences of the skin, has endured to our days.

Ætius enumerates a variety of remedies in use in ancient times, and shows much discernment in his commendation of the best among them.

None of the ancients have proposed a more ridiculous remedy than Marcellus ("Med. Art. Princip.," tom. ii., p. 399). He says, "The best cure for corns occasioned by the friction of the shoe

---

* The Translator has ventured to recommend, instead of the Author's "unguent of *frogs* and *quadrupled mercury*," a simpler and more modern, as well as more efficacious application.—*Tr.*

## EFFECTS OF ILL-MADE SHOES.

is to apply to them the ashes of an old shoe mingled with oil."

Children, and persons of advanced age, women especially, neglect their toe-nails, which then grow and form excrescences like horns. I have seen some which, rising from the great toe, formed a curve that passed over all the other toes. I have seen these horns upon both feet; and upon the second as well as the great toe; all the nails, indeed, are capable of forming such horns, in size proportioned to the size of the toes. I have several curious examples preserved in spirits, and such are to be met with in most anatomical collections. M. de Buffon has described, in the 14th volume of his "Natural History," a nail of a spiral form nearly half a foot long, and having a circumference of nearly two inches. This nail was removed by M. Campenon, from the great toe of a woman seventy-five years of age. It had been twelve years growing to this size.

I have sometimes seen a hard and spongy substance growing under the nails, which raised them up, and projected considerably, not having been meddled with for a long time, for fear of exciting inflammation. I have removed it successfully, after the nail had been softened in warm water, when it can be gradually cut away without pain or danger.

When the nails are very long and hard, they should be carefully scraped, and then cut with a sharp knife.

I will now conclude my observations upon the best form of shoes and boots; and the reader may judge for himself whether this subject, which appears at the first glance of such small importance, does not deserve to be treated with attention and respect. He may then pass judgment upon Posidonius, who declared, " that the art of shoemaking was most probably invented and perfected by philosophers."

# PART II.

# THE HUMAN FOOT,

## AND ITS COVERING.

### BY JAMES DOWIE.

"To know
That which before us lies in daily life
Is the prime wisdom."—*Milton.*

"'Tis the sublime of man,
Our noontide majesty, to know ourselves,
Parts and proportions of a wondrous whole."—*Coleridge.*

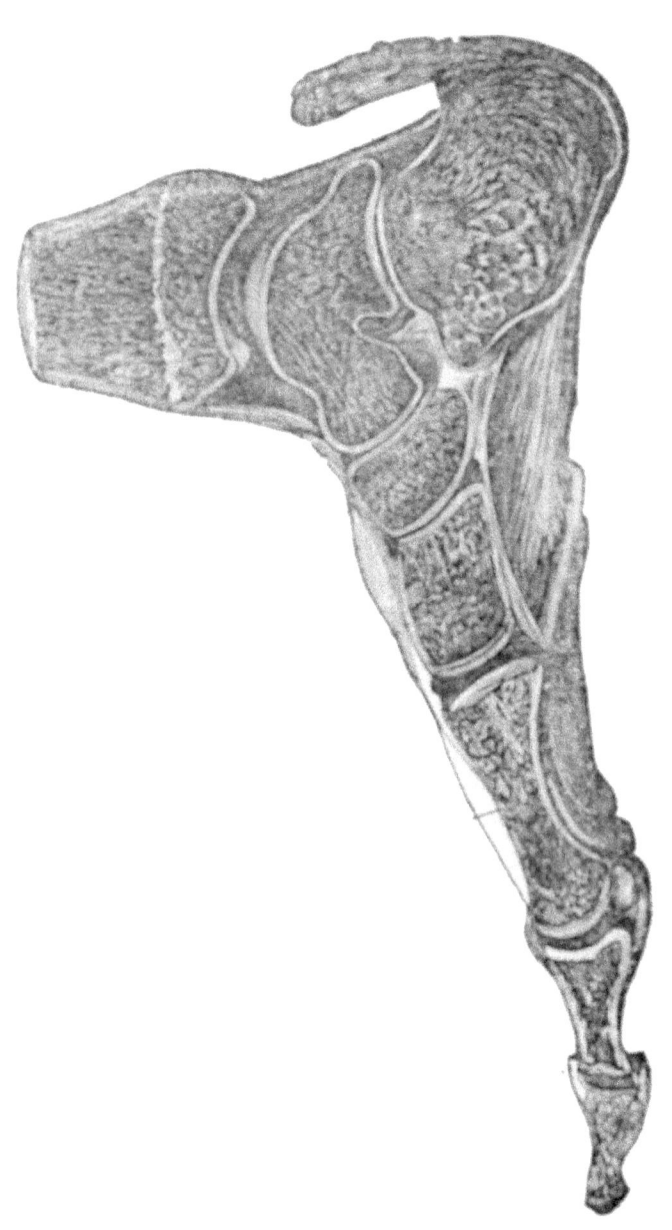

# THE FOOT, AND ITS COVERING.

## CHAPTER I.

INTRODUCTION.

1. It would be superfluous in me to advance a single sentence in support of the inestimable value of Dr. Camper's Essay on the "Best Form of Shoe," almost every word of which is applicable to the present state of things. It was a firm conviction of its importance in the cause of progress that induced me to give the preceding translation, and I flatter myself it will be the means of stimulating the further investigation of the subject it treats, in accordance with the wishes of its celebrated author.

2. On comparing Dr. Camper's work with a Paper read before the Royal Scottish Society of Arts in 1839,* by me, a very remarkable coincidence of opinion will be found expressed, considering the

* Published in the Society's Select Transactions for March, 1839, and the "Edinburgh New Philosophical Journal," No. 52.

difference of circumstances under which the two were written, both advocating the same cause, with nearly the same arguments, and consequently arriving at similar conclusions.

3. The only difference between the two works meriting notice in this place is *Elasticated leather* (an article invented since the date of Dr. Camper's work), and its adaptation to the purpose for which it was invented—a purpose in which it has now been successfully employed for upwards of twenty years.

4. The real object apparently sought by Dr. Camper manifests itself to be involved in the difference just noticed (3).* This is all but proved to a demonstration by the fact that, throughout the whole of his work he objects, in the strongest terms, to rigid material for the construction of shoes—no less soles than uppers; his advocacy from first to last being leather of a quality to meet the contraction and elongation of muscle.

5. I also treat, perhaps, somewhat more prominently, the elongation of the foot under the pressure of the weight of the body when in an erect position or attitude, as in walking. Medical men are familiar with this elongation; but they are not, apparently, sensible of the extent for which provision should be made in the construction of the sole of the boot or

* The figures within parenthesis throughout the work refer to the sections, unless otherwise specified.

shoe. Of this more after (76), when I come to discuss the requirements of the human foot; at present I merely draw attention to a characteristic difference which exists between the two works, in reference to the flattening of the arch of the foot under pressure, and its consequent elongation (27).

6. The author's Paper referred to above (2) was got up at the request of his friends, purposely to draw attention to his patent elastic boots and shoes, which were at the time beginning to be extensively approved and worn by some of the most distinguished citizens of Edinburgh. It was read before the Society of Arts with a view to procure their patronage as a scientific body interested in all improvements in applied science, and this was unanimously granted, with more than ordinary approbation, as will be seen from their Journal. On this occasion the patent elastic boot itself was exhibited to the members present, and more attention was of course paid to its manufacture than to the writing of the Paper; in short, the object of the lecture was merely to give just such a general outline of the subject as to provoke the public discussion of the elastic principle.

7. From the Paper being thus wanting in many respects relative to detail, a strong demand has been made upon the author for the present work, some of his best customers and friends, since the expiry of his patent (his invention now being public property),

having been more than ordinarily solicitous at times for something more being said about elasticated leather, and its adaptation to the wants of the lower extremities, more especially in reference to the elastic principle involved in my proposition; as much as to say that I had not given in my specification sufficient publicity to the object of my invention, in accordance with the spirit of the Patent Laws; and that, consequently, I still owed a debt to the public—"a final dividend," as they say, "to make full payment,"—urging their plea by many arguments "that such a work was required," and that "it should be written by a practical man."

8. But writing books is hardly compatible with my profession as a shoemaker. At the same time, it must be granted that every Practice has its Science, and that the shoemaker is in duty bound to contribute to the advancement of the latter, as well as to the improvement of the former—the proposition of St. Crispin being no exception to the common rule of progress.

9. In responding to demands of this kind, scientific readers will, in this place, pardon the expression of a hope that a liberal allowance be made to the pen of a practical man, who feels conscious of having much to apologize for, even on the very threshold of his task. The subject is truly, in all its branches, one of progress, involving many intricate questions in science, some of which are not yet more

## INTRODUCTION.

than sufficiently understood for practical application. But the traveller cannot always suspend his journey on the approach of night, so that when he stumbles and falls, he must just rise again, shake himself, and make the best of a trackless road he can, until break of day. So is it with the manufacture of boots and shoes, and the materials of which they are made : for if the advance since Dr. Camper's time is behind the general progress of things, that is only the best and most cogent of reasons for the shoemaker and the leather trade generally doubling their diligence for the future.

10. The customers' view of the subject is decidedly of a kindred character. The prevalence of corns, bunions, distortions, and like deformities, prove this in so forcible a manner that few will ask for more satisfactory evidence in support of the truth of the general proposition, that every one who wears a boot or a shoe has a duty to perform in the cause of progress, as well as an interest to defend ; for unless boots and shoes are worn, who can estimate their value, or measure the advance made in the march of improvement ?

11. The grand consideration in the manufacture of a boot or shoe is the physical well-being of the foot. This is a proposition so self-evident, that its enunciation may appear, at first sight, superfluous ; but when the facts of the case at issue are examined from a practical point of view, the reverse will be

found true ;—for how often is the comfort of the foot sacrificed at the shrine of fashion, or in compliance with some pennywise and pound foolish notion equally disastrous in its consequences? Indeed, in practice, the question just stands thus: " Better off the feet than out of the fashion ! " How few, it may be fairly asked, are there whose feet have not been less or more injured by improperly constructed boots and shoes! Few indeed, and far between, are the feet that display their natural beauty, and perform with anything like comparative freedom their natural functions according to the design of the All-wise Creator!

12. "PRACTICE with SCIENCE" is the motto of the Royal Agricultural Society, and why should it not be St. Crispin's golden rule? It is certainly high time that its spirit were adopted in the trade, and that routine, fashion, and everything else in the manufacture of boots and shoes were made subservient to the structure and physical well-being of the foot. In the olden time it was said, that "Socrates brought philosophy from the clouds," and Dr. Camper's essay on the "BEST FORM OF SHOE" is acknowledged by its talented author as a condescension from the philosopher's chair. The writer of this, on the contrary, has hitherto fought his way upwards from *the last*, and the longer he investigates his subject the more he finds it necessary to attend to this rule,—one which is simply the maxim of the above Society, the leading foot in the march of

progress being that of experience, the only sure foundation upon which a solid superstructure can be built in any of the arts.

13. The subject of the work, it will thus be seen, involves a two-fold consideration, the *first* being the foot, and the *second* its covering, including the stocking as well as the boot or shoe; so that it will be necessary to examine the mechanical structure of the former, its physical well-being and requirements, under the various circumstances in which it is placed in the struggle of life, before we proceed to the discussion of the latter.

## CHAPTER II.

### ON THE EXTERNAL ANATOMY OF THE FOOT, FROM A SHOEMAKER'S POINT OF VIEW.

14. It is said that "no two faces are alike," and the same thing may almost be affirmed of feet. To appearance, and even according to the ordinary mode of measurement, differences may be found extremely small in many cases ; but when the question of "a proper fit" is raised, then, however small and apparently insignificant such differences may be, they require the closest attention of the shoemaker to provide for the well-being of the foot.

15. In every case "a proper fit" is an individual question. The shoemaker may take one view of this question, it may be, and his customers another ; but removed from the sphere of opinion, self-interest, fashion, and prejudice, it involves simply a covering of such a character as will provide for the physical wellbeing of the foot, under all the circumstances in which it is placed.

16. What, then, is the nature of this covering ? Age, occupation, summer and winter, latitude, and the like, advance their respective claims for consideration ; but before these can be successfully investi-

gated, it will be necessary to notice from a general point of view the peculiar form and mechanism of the foot.

17. The form of the foot is ever changing with the different positions which it occupies in walking, its form in one position being different from its form in another. The foot of a statue is uniform—so is the foot of a man in a state of rest, waiving the question of temperature, circulation of the blood, &c.; but when walking it occupies an ever-varying position, while in a corresponding manner it is continually changing its form.

18. The measurement of the foot is thus in one position or attitude different from what it is in another—measurement in repose, for example, the attitude in which it is generally taken, being different from measurement taken while the foot is in motion, as in walking, or under pressure.

19. The differences of measurement, and consequently of form, just noticed (17 and 18), arise from the peculiar functions the foot has to perform in the grand mechanical system which the body as a living organism exemplifies in progression or other movement where the mobility of its parts is displayed (25).

20. Dr. Camper has drawn attention to some of those functions, principally from an anatomical point of view; but from their importance to the shoemaker, successful locomotion being almost entirely dependent upon their proper performance, it will be necessary to

notice them somewhat more fully from a mechanical point of view, in order to comprehend how far they are interfered with by different kinds of boots and shoes, what are the movements the foot actually performs, and also, what is the real nature of the covering the lower extremities require.

21. The legs and feet in walking form together a compound system of levers; the ground under the latter is the fulcrum to this system; the weight moved is the body, and any burden it may carry; the motive power is partly gravitation and partly muscular force;—while the object of boots and shoes is to prevent the fulcrum end of the system sustaining harm, affording it, at the same time, free action.

22. Examined in detail, almost every bone forms a lever—every joint or articulation a fulcrum—every contracting muscle a force; while the resistance to be overcome includes, not only the weight of the body and its locomotion through space and the atmosphere, but the action of antagonistic muscles in the performance of their respective functions.

23. The movements in walking barefoot on a level surface may be thus described. In starting from a state of repose in an erect attitude, and leading off with the right foot, the first thing done is gently to throw the whole of the weight of the body upon the left foot. As soon as the right foot is thus relieved, it leads off, the right leg being stretched forward, while the foot is being at the same time extended by the con-

traction of the muscles of the calf of the leg and sole of the foot, so that the sole as it advances remains nearly parallel to the ground. On the right leg and foot being thus extended, the centre of gravity is by the force of other muscles of the body also gradually thrown forward, while the heel of the left foot, by this and the contraction of the muscles of the calf of the leg and sole of the foot, is raised from the ground, and the whole weight of the body for a moment of time placed upon the toes of that foot (the left one), such being now the point of the system of leverage that rests upon the ground (*i. e.*, the fulcrum). From this point the weight is now thrown forward upon the right foot in a manner that produces nearly uniform progression, as will subsequently be shown (161 and 203), when the system enjoys unrestrained freedom. The centre of gravity of action being thus gradually brought forward over the right foot, the left foot at the same time being raised from the ground, it is then moved past the right leg, when it is next extended; and thus progression is effected, step by step, the force and centre of gravity moving in a sort of zigzag line from foot to foot—this alternate divergence from rectilinear motion being greater in woman than in man, and in broad, fat men than in those whose form and corpulence is the reverse: altogether the movements of the foot in walking are very interesting.

24. Such is but a very cursory and imperfect view

of the mechanical details involved in pedestrian exercise, so necessary for the health of the foot and the system generally; but imperfect as it is, it will be sufficient to enable us to examine the functions of the foot relative to the different forms and measurements which it exhibits, and also the nature of the covering it consequently requires. The best illustration is for every one to examine his own foot and leg in walking, as subsequently noticed (69, 70, and 201), for if this is done, the facts of the case under consideration cannot fail to be realized in a manner that will satisfy the reader as to their paramount importance.

25. I have now to examine the elongation of the foot, in order to account for those differences of form and measurement exemplified in walking, alluded to in a previous section (19).

26. The elongation of the foot in walking, on a level surface, is of a twofold character. In both, it is very different in different forms of feet, as will subsequently be shown (36 and 37). In this place, observation will be confined to the two ways under which elongation takes place.

27. When the weight of the body is thrown upon the arch of the foot, as in standing or walking, its elongation is effected by the flattening of the arch and the consequent receding of the toes from the heel; the process of lengthening thus taking place backwards as well as forwards. It has already been shown

in Dr. Camper's work (Part I., p. 13) that the bones of the foot are so tied and braced together by means of ligaments, tendons, and muscles, as to form an elastic arch, like the spring of a carriage—that the weight of the body pressing upon the crown of this arch, flattens it in the same manner as the weight of the carriage, with its contents, flattens its springs, the two ends of which recede from each other as the centre is pressed down. In like manner the heel recedes from the toes by the flattening of the instep, so that the distance between them increases; in other words, the length of the foot increases as its arch is flattened.

28. When the whole weight of the body is thrown upon one foot with the momentum due to the rate of progression, as we have seen is the case in walking (23), the flattening of the arch and elongation of that foot must be considerable. It will be still more so in running than in walking, and in jumping than in running. Other examples of a kindred character are seen in going down hill, down stairs, &c. &c. (38, 39, and 40.)

29. The second kind of elongation of the sole of the foot takes place at the articulation of the bones of the toes with those of the metatarsus, when the toes turn upwards. The cause of this increase of length is the turning of the toes upon the metatarsal bones on the principle of a hinge; so that, were the bend of the great toe with the first metatarsus a

right angle, then the increase of length would be equal to the thickness of the joint. It is different in different individuals, whose feet are differently arched ; but in every case is equal to the elongation of the muscles of the sole of the foot, to which must be added the distance the heel-bone is pulled towards the toes, when the metatarsus is brought nearly into the line of the leg.

30. When the toes are turned upwards, while the heel and forepart of the metatarsal bones are resting upon the ground, then the elongation of the sole takes place at the toes. In other words, the points of the toes recede from the bottom upwards more than their length by the thickness of the joint, supposing a right angle made. In proof of this, put the foot upon a slip of paper or other measure exactly its own length, then, without raising the tarsus and metatarsus, turn up the great toe, when it will be found to advance considerably beyond the length of the paper.

31. But when the toes rest upon the ground, remaining in this position for a time stationary, as they do in walking (23), then the tarsus turns upwards ; the elongation thus taking place backwards towards the heel. Proof of this may also be effected by a strip of paper, or measuring-line, as before (30).

32. This elongation backwards is in some measure compensated by the heel turning downwards, the extremity of the heel-bone being pulled a little

forward towards the bend of the great toe by the muscles of the sole, the arch of the foot being thus increased in height, while its span is consequently reduced in length. The amount of this compensation is different in different forms of the heel, but is never equal to the total elongation of the foot backwards; that is to say, the length of the sole from the point of the great toe to the extremity of the heel, when thus bent upwards, exceeds the length of the sole when straight and in a state of repose, there being no pressure upon the arch of the foot to flatten it. The reason of this will readily be understood when it is observed that the metatarsus is brought nearly into line with the leg, so that the distance between the ball of the great toe and calf of the leg round the heel is shortened.

33. The bones of the foot form a double arch, being arched longitudinally and laterally, or lengthways and sideways. This arises in consequence of the span from the heel to the lenticular bone, or fore-end of the first metatarsal bone, being higher and longer than the span from the heel to the fore-end of the fifth metatarsal bone, where it articulates with the little toe. This latter arch is so low that, when covered with muscle and skin, the outside of the foot, from the heel to the little toe, touches the ground in walking in very many cases, if not the majority; the tarsus and metatarsus thus forming an irregularly-shaped portion of a dome.

34. From this dome-like peculiarity of structure, the foot, it will thus be seen, when under pressure, expands from the heel laterally and longitudinally in the direction of the little toe, as well as longitudinally from the heel in the direction of the great toe, as pointed out in previous sections (27 and 28).

35. This peculiar double-arched structure of the foot, subject to longitudinal and latter expansion, greatly increases its strength and stability, without diminishing its elasticity. As Holden justly observes, in his work on "Human Osteology," if the foot had been composed "only of a single bone, like a shoemaker's last, how much more liable it would have been to fracture and dislocation!" and, it may be added, the less the longitudinal and lateral expansion of the foot, the more liable is it to such injuries. In other words, if this longitudinal and lateral expansion is prevented by improperly-constructed boots and shoes, as subsequently shown (167—176), then the foot will thereby become liable to fracture, distortion, dislocation, and other maladies of a kindred character.

36. Longitudinal expansion is greatest in long, high-arched, slender feet; and least in short, low-arched, strong, thick feet.

37. Lateral expansion, again, is greatest in high-arched, broad feet; and least in low-arched, narrow ones.

38. There is another peculiar characteristic of the

arch of the foot that demands attention, viz., the elasticity or flattening of the instep in throwing the weight of the body from one foot on to another. The expansion of the arch in this case, it will be perceived, takes place only on one side, and is the reverse of what is effected on the opposite at the tarsus, for the heel bends downwards and inwards, thus increasing the depth of the arch (32), and reducing the length of its span; but at the instep an opposite effect is produced, the flattening of this portion of the arch diminishing its depth, but increasing its span. In running, going up hill, or up and down stairs, the fore part of the arch of the foot is thus subjected to considerable strain, and, but for its elasticity, would suffer harm, or the pedestrian would be obliged to adopt strategical means, as in the case of a flat foot, subsequently shown (190), and also through rigid-soled boots and shoes (175 and 190).

39. In going down a steep hill, or any steep incline, as the roof of a house, the heel end of the arch has to bear the extra strain, one of the most trying positions of the foot, because mechanically the weakest. It is on this account that so many sprains at the ankle are sustained in running incautiously down-hill by those not accustomed to such pedestrian feats. In those accustomed to climb and descend steep inclines, as shepherds in mountainous sheep walks, the muscles, tendons, and ligaments of the

foot acquire by exercise increased strength to meet the extra strain upon them, in a similar manner to the often quoted case of the arms of the blacksmith, or St. Crispin's thumbs.

40. The greater strain upon the muscles, tendons, and ligaments of the foot and leg experienced in going down stairs, than in going up, may be thus explained. In going upstairs, the instep has only to sustain the weight of the body while the other foot is being raised the exact height of a step, so that by adding step to step the sum or total height to which the body is raised from the bottom to the top of the stair, is attained without loss; but on coming down so much has to be added to each step, while the foot is in a weaker position to sustain this extra strain. This arises from the body having to be raised up upon the toes at every step in going down, under the hypothesis that the heel is allowed to touch the step at every descent, a result but too common. Under such circumstances, the heel is first raised, and the weight of the body placed upon the toes of the foot that rests upon the step. The other foot then descends, and receives the whole of the weight of the body upon it when placed flat upon the next step, from a higher level than that of the step from which it descended, so that the sum of the ascents has to be added to the total height of the stair. Moreover, in turning upon the edge of the step as a fulcrum, the toes, instep, ancle, and knee

are in the weakest attitude to sustain the force of this weight, so that the unfavourable position of the muscles, tendons, and ligaments under such circumstances will readily be seen; and when I come to apply the *data* here involved to the case of millers and others, who have to carry heavy loads up and down stairs (91), and who are often obliged to go down back foremost or sideways, or lean to the handrail, my readers will perceive how far it bears upon the manufacture of boots and shoes. The data thus advanced also account for the comparative ease with which those having healthy strong feet go downstairs, such as waiters in hotels, for in going down they never let the heel touch the step at all, but descend from toe to toe as it were, taking full advantage of the elasticity of the instep—the centre of gravity, descending uniformly nearly in a straight line, instead of rising so much at every step against the downward momentum and gravity of the body, as we shall see in the case of sufferers from corns, bunions, and rigid-soled boots and shoes, when we come to that division of the work (Chap. XI.).

41. The form and position of the great toe next claim consideration. This part of the foot has special functions to perform, and consequently demands a corresponding amount of attention from the shoemaker before he can protect it from injury, and keep it in thorough working order and usefulness. It involves, in walking and running, as has

been shown (23), that point upon which not only the whole weight of the body is placed, but which also has to sustain the muscular thrust required to propel this weight from one foot to another throughout the fatiguing length of many a long journey, consequently it is that point of the grand system of leverage resting on the fulcrum (*i. e.*, the ground) around which the momenta have to be taken, in estimating the value of whatever progression is made. It is the axle of the fly-wheel, as it were, upon the truthfulness of whose revolutions centres are easily crossed without harm, and the regular motion of the several parts preserved economically and successfully, without a break-down, throughout the entire length of the journey. Such is a general view of the dependance of man upon the proper discharge of the functions of his great toe in walking, and which, when not discharged, give rise to a fresh start at every step, and consequently to a jolting gait, with a heavy waste of motive power (muscular force). But more of this in its proper place afterwards (158).

42. The peculiar forms and positions of the great toe that chiefly claim attention of the shoemaker, are thickness at the point, length, and direction, as to whether the axis of the toe runs in a straight line with the axis of the first metatarsal bone, so as to make the inside of the foot straight from heel to toe.

43. As to thickness at the point, two extremes

and a mean may be taken to illustrate the principles involved. In one, the foot at the great toe tapers gradually from the metatarsal joint or instep, to the point terminating in what may be called a blunt wedge. In the other extreme—that which gives the shoemaker most concern and trouble—the toe is thicker at the point than at the middle or first joint, the wedge in this case being reversed, back foremost. In another chapter (XI.) we shall find, that a very large number of this class of toes, especially when they are long, suffer an extreme amount of misery from disease of various kinds, arising from improper coverings. Of the mean between these two extremes nothing need be said in this place.

44. As to the length of the great toe, two extremes and a mean may also be taken to illustrate principle. In the one extreme, both the toe and its metatarsus are short, the joint being not much in advance of that of the little toe. In the other extreme, the reverse of this is the case, the toe and its metatarsus being both long, and the bending of the foot at the toes more oblique. The mean examples in this case are considerably diversified, owing to the length of the toe and the length of its metatarsus being both involved.

45. As Dr. Camper observes, the second toe is generally longer than the first. But the shoemaker's question is, the thickness of the toes and the form which they give to this part of the foot. Three ex-

amples may again be given to illustrate this two extremes and a mean.

46. When the foot at the root of the toes is broad, flat, and the toes long, as shown Plate III., Fig. 4, the greatest care is necessary to preserve them in their natural position through infancy and youth, so as to have a healthy, useful foot in after-life. Among half-civilized and barefooted tribes, healthy feet of this class are common; but among the civilized nations of the world, examples are few and far between. The reason is this — the length of the toe gives greater leverage to the wedging process of forcing a broad foot into a narrow-toed boot or shoe, as seen in the example quoted, 187, and to which we refer, and also 243.

47. In the other extreme the toes form a more acute angle in front, being what is termed "narrow." The expression narrow, however, is often not a very correct one, the toes being actually, when individually considered, thicker than those of the other extreme; but from being articulated more obliquely to the metatarsal bones, the joints have more room, owing to the one being behind the other, and therefore are different when thus individually considered. Nevertheless, collectively, viewing the toes the foot is narrow. The mean between the two extremes requires no notice.

48. A well-formed foot in middle life is generally straight from heel to toe on the inside. In infancy,

however, the point of the great toe projects outwards from the other toes, so that at this period the inside of the foot forms a curve, or is concave. This is owing to the peculiar state of the tarsal bones, and of the muscles, tendons, and ligaments of the toes and instep at this tender age, so that the spreading of the toes, and the narrowness of the tarsus are wise provisions in the feet of children to meet their sprawling about in learning to walk, and to promote the healthy development of the whole. In old age there is an opposite tendency from that of childhood, owing to the enlargement of the tarsal bones, the sinking of the lateral arch, and the increase of thickness that takes place below the ankle—these changes giving to the inside of the foot a convex form; while, to increase this natural convexity, the great toe is too often turned inwards at the point by an improper covering.

49. The peculiar arched construction of the foot, with its elastic lateral and longitudinal expansion, forwards in front when walking, running, or leaping, and backwards behind, merits a special notice, as no other arrangement of parts could, from the erect position and weight of the body of man, have prevented his foot from sustaining fracture and dislocation. Altogether the design is a perfect masterpiece which claims from every intelligent mind the highest degree of admiration. Sometimes the production of man's handicraft will bear a superficial

examination, at other times hardly so much; but the more closely the internal and external anatomy of the foot is examined, the more satisfied is the mind with the wisdom of its GREAT CREATOR, as displayed in the perfection of its design; and with the duty incumbent upon all of attending with religious propriety and respect to the natural development of its parts, and to the healthy performance of all its functions. Had the arch been of longitudinal construction only, it could not have sustained the lateral thrust from the momentum of the body in its zigzag line from foot to foot (23). We could not even have walked upon a carpeted floor with safety and ease; but the lateral arch makes provision for this zigzag exigency in the roughest road the foot of man has to encounter in his journey through the uneven and rugged wilderness of this world.

50. The foot exemplifies a considerable diversity of this longitudinal and lateral curvature and expansibility, better known, perhaps, by the form of the instep. Three examples may again be given in illustration of principle—two extremes and a mean.

51. Some insteps rise very high, are finely arched, but narrow above, and do not fill the measure well.

52. The opposite extreme is nearly a flat foot, the lateral and longitudinal arches being low, and the girth small, the instep being flat both above and below.

53. The mean between these two extremes is a

medium arch, well rounded transversely above, and girths more than either of the other two examples.

54. The projection of the heelbone next demands attention. It is often very different in different individuals. In some races, as Indians, it is said to be very prominent; but let differences be great or small, they all require the special attention of the shoemaker, no less for the girth of the ankle than the position of the leg of the boot or the tie of the shoe. The principal characteristic which claims his chiefest attention, however, is the peculiar leverage involved in the action of the muscles of the back of the leg and sole of the foot, whose tendons are attached to the heelbone, the contraction of these muscles increasing the length of the radius of the leg, as seen in the case of walking (23, 27, and 201).

55. There is a similar diversity of the ankle, a joint which requires special consideration, not so much in reference to the girth of the leg at this articulation, as to the fact that the joint itself is a most important fulcrum in many of the principal movements of the foot in progression; consequently the joint, with its ligaments, tendons, and muscles, ought to possess in the boot or shoe that freedom of action so essentially necessary to preserve its physical well-being when in a healthy state and unrestrained by its coverings, which it naturally possesses (see Chap. III.).

56. The projection of the heelbone and peculiarities of the ankle, depend as much, perhaps, upon

the form and position of the astragalus as upon that of the heelbone itself. In other words, the length to which the heelbone projects backwards depends upon the form of the arch and the point in that arch upon which the bone of the leg rests. Different examples of projection and setting on of the leg upon the arch, in this respect, give rise just to as many different propositions in the manufacture of a boot or shoe.

57. The muscles, tendons, ligaments, grooves, sheaths, and other apparatus of this kind in which they work, may not inaptly be termed *the foot tackle*, or the tackling of the ship; and, unless kept in proper working trim, the ship will become unmanageable, and consequently be liable to founder in any sudden squall, while even in fine weather and smooth sailing the general wear and tear upon the tackle will be greatly increased. The diameter of the pulleys, the length and size of the ropes, and the angles at which they pull and are pulled, are all very different in the feet of some individuals from what they are in those of others, and even in the same foot when in different positions, every case requiring the greatest circumspection to preserve its physical well-being.

## CHAPTER III.

### THE PHYSICAL WELL-BEING OF THE FOOT.

58. THE object of the covering being to protect the foot from injury, the sanitary condition of its mechanism, or the maintaining the foot in a healthy state, will briefly be examined in this chapter. In a subsequent one (Chap. XI.) the restoration of diseased feet to a sound condition will be investigated, so far as a cure can be effected by the covering ; but as " prevention is better than cure," it will be advisable to consider separately in this place the former question.

59. The general question, that upon the physical well-being of the foot no small amount of the health of the whole system depends, first demands notice. Its truth is so universally acknowledged as to render anything more than the enunciation of the proposition superfluous.

60. But although experience has extorted from mankind in general a sort of tacit consent to the truth of the proposition, that a sympathetic relationship exists between the foot and the lungs and other vital parts ; that sad consequences arise from wet feet, cold feet, corns, bunions, and the long catalogue

of malformations when improper coverings are worn; yet there appears to be a blind submission to these things, as if they were the common lot of fallen humanity! Savages wear large pegs in their lips, mould their heads into a flat or square form, and follow other barbarous practices peculiar to savage life; but it is certainly humiliating to think that civilized England should pursue a similar course towards the lower extremities of her offspring.

61. This no doubt arises, it will perhaps be said, in some measure, from the little progress made by my profession in that department of science to which this work belongs, owing, as I have already said, in no small degree, to the many unsettled questions involved relative to the daily tear and wear or waste upon the foot, and the reformative process of repairing its peculiar structure.

62. But although many points in this department of applied science may not yet be acknowledged as settled, it is, nevertheless, a well-authenticated fact that the daily waste upon the foot, however it may take place, and whatever may be the peculiar results it gives rise to in different constitutions, is considerable, even in the best state of health; that this waste is largely given off between the toes, as well as from the surface of the foot generally; that walking in badly-fitting stockings and shoes greatly increases its daily amount; and that, in extreme cases, in warm weather, both feet and stockings

PHYSICAL WELL-BEING OF THE FOOT. 75

smell so strongly as to be intolerable when the boot or shoe is taken off, even in cases where the stockings are daily changed and the feet washed and kept clean.

63. But although exercise with an improper covering increases the daily waste, yet it is an equally well-established fact, that exercise is also essentially necessary to a healthy organism, and nowhere is this more imperatively true than in the bones, ligaments, tendons, and muscles of the foot. This arises from the extra work they have to perform in supporting the weight of the body, and in effecting its locomotion. If we stop but for a moment to estimate this weight, and the manner it is transported over a long journey in walking, it will readily be seen that the tear and wear upon the foot-tackle must of necessity be very great—that the amount of daily waste given off must consequently be great also—and that no other sort of material could endure the strain upon it but the living foot-tackle itself. Now, if the tear and wear is great, the building-up must correspond, to maintain an equilibrium; otherwise the tackle becomes subject to atrophy or wasting. But if this removal of the daily waste and the reformative process of building up cannot be effected without exercise, it naturally follows that the first thing to be attended to is the free action of the bones, ligaments, tendons, and muscles of the foot in walking or other exercise to which it is subject. In the language of Sir C.

Bell, "The foot has an internal play which should be preserved."

64. It is therefore with the external form of the foot the shoemaker has to deal, and its internal mechanism or tackle only so far as it affects outward form. The *rationale* of this will readily be seen; for if provision is made for the outside, the inside will also be provided for, so far, at least, as regards that freedom of action upon which its healthy structure depends.

65. Exercise, so far as it lies within the province of the shoemaker, is simply in the shoeing of man, to preserve for his foot the perfect freedom of all its functions. If the bones, ligaments, tendons, muscles, nerves, and arteries have the same freedom of play within the covering that they have when he is walking barefoot, then they will receive that amount of exercise necessary to health. But if, on the contrary, they, or any one or more of them, are so interfered with by the stocking, boot, or shoe, as to prevent their natural freedom of action, then disease in some form or other must of necessity be sooner or later experienced.

66. Of the various diseases to which the foot of man is subject, and which can generally be prevented by a proper covering, it will be sufficient for illustration if we mention weakness of the ankle, instep, toes, &c. as belonging to one class, and corns, bunions, inflamed joints, &c. as belonging to another.

67. When a customer enters the shop, and gives his order for the first time, stating the kind and quality of the article wanted, the first thing the shoemaker has to attend to, is the healthy character of his foot. Inquiry into this takes precedence of inquiry as to size and peculiar form, because the necessary information regarding the former is, in the generality of cases, more difficult to be acquired, than that regarding the latter. He sees at a glance if it is a narrow or a broad foot—a long or a short one—a flat foot or one high in the instep; and whether the heel projects far behind, or is nearly perpendicular. All these are perceptible to the eye, and subject to measurement; but when he begins to handle, and comes first to one corn, then another, and so on to bunions, inflamed joints, and other unseen deformities, for which provision has to be made, he not unfrequently meets, at the same time, a disposition on the part of his customer to conceal half the truth, if not something more, relative to these things, a general indifference being manifested to the sanitary condition of the feet. Customers have, doubtless, a right to put their own value upon their own feet; but in the shoeing, it is certainly far from a wise economy to conceal anything for which special provision has to be made by their shoemaker.

68. It is the healthy foot, however, that is now under investigation, with a view to preserve it in all

its integrity as to muscular elasticity and strength. It is a well-known fact, one with which all are familiar, that muscular strength may be cultivated—that it is capable of being greatly raised above what may be termed its normal or conservative standard. The hands and arms of the blacksmith is an oft-quoted example of this kind, as already noticed. The feet of the rope-dancer and of all who like him take much exercise in *thin* shoes, where the muscles of the feet have their free and natural play, is another illustration more immediately applicable to our subject. Now, successful cases like these exemplify, in a very forcible manner, the simple but efficacious means at the command of every one, rich and poor, for the improvement of the feet—means for keeping them, not merely in a normal state of health and strength, but in the enjoyment of something better—art, as it were, providing the means for enabling Nature to advance herself from a comparative to a superlative degree of health and strength.

69. The means which improve the physical wellbeing of the foot, cultivate, at the same time, the general health of the body. There is thus a harmony of design exemplified throughout the whole system not undeserving of attention; for the means of health is exercise in walking, which calls into play not merely the muscles, tendons, ligaments, and bones of the feet, but those of the whole body, every

function and faculty of body and *mind* being engaged. To satisfy ourselves of the truth of this, we have only, in walking through the room with the boots or shoes off, so as to give the feet every freedom of action, to grasp the legs with the hands, when the muscles below the knee will be found in an active state. If the hands are removed to the thighs, the hip-joint, or the lumbar region, the same active state of the muscles is experienced; the chest, top of the shoulder, the neck, and even the crown of the head, are also all less or more called into motion by the simple exercise of walking. When a child begins to walk, it moves its arms at the same time that it moves its legs, thus illustrating, in a very interesting manner, not only the equilibrium of posture, but also the sympathetic relation that exists between the different members of the body—a relation that is preserved throughout the whole period of life, from infancy to old age. Paley, referring to posture in infancy, says:—

"A child learning to walk is the greatest posture-master in the world; but art, if it may be so called, sinks into habit, and he is soon able to poise himself in a great variety of attitudes, without being sensible either of caution or effort. But still there must be an aptitude of parts upon which habit can thus attach,—a previous capacity of motions which the animal is thus taught to exercise; and the facility with which this exercise is acquired, forms one object of our admiration. What parts are principally employed, or in what manner each contributes to its office, is difficult to explain. Perhaps the obscure motion of the bones of the feet may have their share in this effect. They are put in motion by every slip or vacillation of the body, and seem to assist in restoring its balance. Certain it is, that this circumstance in the structure of the foot, and by its being composed of many small bones, applied to and articulating with one another, by diversely-shaped surfaces, instead of being made of one piece, like the last of a shoe, is very remarkable. I suppose also that it would be difficult to stand firmly upon stilts or wooden legs, though their base exactly imitated the figure and dimensions of the sole of the foot."

70. Again, if we suspend for a moment the muscular functions of the foot, so as to render, as it were, the tarsus, metatarsus, and toes one rigid body, like a shoemaker's last, and then walk through the room, it will be found, on examining the legs, thighs, and other parts, as before (69), that we thus, by this rigidity of the feet, arrest, as it were, with the hand of Death, half the health-giving agency of the system. We not only do so, but we, at the same time, impose a greater amount of work upon the locomotive tackle of the legs and feet now called into play than it is able to bear, thus rendering the very exercise of walking a painful wasting process instead of a sanitary blessing !

71. The practical study of pedestrian exercise, with a view to the physical well-being of the foot, is thus an interesting one to all who have any regard for their general health. It involves many important considerations for a thinking public ; for when the foot is neglected in infancy and youth, the after-

period of life experiences a saddening amount of suffering, from persons being unable to take the necessary amount of exercise that their health requires. How many are there in this great metropolis who contrive by every means in their power to shun walking just because of their feet—their shoe pinching them somewhere or other? During the business part of the day, every short cut possible is taken to avoid that kind of exercise which Nature designed for the physical well-being of their bodies; and when they emerge from the bustle and smoke of the city to the pure air of the suburbs, instead of entertaining the thought of *a health-giving family walk*, the pinching shoe is immediately pulled off and the aching imprisoned feet flung upon the sofa in slippers in search of relief, while the mind but too often finds consolation in attributing the injuries experienced to everything else but the real cause. How different is it with those who have healthy feet, and who are familiar, scientifically as well as practically, with the inestimable blessings arising from the daily exercise in walking or riding in a pure atmosphere.

72. The physical well-being of the foot, in relation to the general health of the body, is now beginning to engage particular attention, not only in this country, but also on the continents of Europe and America. Everywhere, physiological anatomists are pointing to the free action of the foot-tackle as the

real foundation of health, and there cannot be a doubt but its proper development and exercise involve the only system of sanitary science that will bear investigation at the bar of Experience. Other means of health may be necessary, but they follow as only the outriders of this the healthy exercise of the body. Its importance, therefore, cannot be too highly estimated by parents, or too earnestly inculcated by them in the domestic circle, where it not unfrequently happens that the health and happiness of their offspring are bartered for an old shoe. Physically, what can be more valuable than the health of the body? When so much anxiety is everywhere expressed relative to the proper education of the rising generation, surely it is not too much to say that every one ought now thoroughly to understand the normal form, development, functions, and physical well-being of his own feet.

73. The sanitary and volunteer movements, at present engrossing so much public attention, are calculated to arouse increasing inquiry relative to the physical well-being of the foot, and the cultivation of a higher standard of national health and strength, by regular exercise daily in walking and riding. The minds of all classes of society are now so thoroughly enlisted in favour of both these movements, that no obstacle thrown in the way, however great, can possibly, for any length of time, impede their progress. Onward things must move in both cases.

What can stop them? At all our schools and seminaries of education, daily exercise in walking is annually becoming more and more the alpha and omega of juvenile training, as it was in the schools of ancient Greece and Rome, teachers everywhere finding from experience that the healthier pupils are, the more rapid progress they make in the various branches of education. Riding-masters, too, are on the increase, and more generally employed by those who can afford exercise on horseback. And although rifle-shooting at the " bull's-eye," with a little "military parade" and "marching out" occasionally, are the chief attractions of the volunteer movement as yet; it nevertheless follows, as a matter of certainty, from the very nature of the tactics involved in the defence of the country by means of the rifle, that the muscular energy of the feet and legs must be attended to, as upon them success will mainly depend, should ever invasion and defence become realities. But the grand realization of the present is the improved state of physical and mental well-being which both these movements have in view.

74. The individual question involved in the physical well-being of the foot is, however, always the most interesting one, because it is everybody's question. It is for everybody, therefore, to think of his or her own foot, and the best means of preserving its health. "Self-preservation is the first law of

Nature;" so that it becomes the duty of all—old and young, rich and poor—to think in accordance with this law of the nature of the covering required by their feet, under the different circumstances and vocations in which they may respectively be placed.

## CHAPTER IV.

INQUIRY INTO THE NATURE OF THE COVERING REQUIRED BY THE HUMAN FOOT, AT DIFFERENT AGES, AND IN DIFFERENT OCCUPATIONS, AND CLIMATES.

75. HAVING in the two preceding chapters considered the ever-varying form, elastic movements, and physical wellbeing of the foot, we are now in a position practically to inquire into the nature of the covering it requires at different ages and in different occupations and climates.

76. From the contractility, expansibility, and mobility of the different parts of the foot considered in relation to one another as living members of one grand system subject to all the changes of organic life, it is very evident that its covering, including the stocking, as well as the boot and shoe, must correspond in elasticity and mobility, each part of the latter harmonizing with its corresponding part of the former. In other words, stockings, boots, and shoes require to be manufactured of elastic materials, to meet the requirements of the human foot.

77. In support of this proposition (76), the following negative proof may be advanced, viz.:—Were the foot shod with cast iron, the shoe having two

side wings, and were it attached to the leg by means of them, and then made fast, as the engineer shoes the fulcrum end of his rocking lever, or as an old naval or military pensioner shoes his wooden leg, the result in walking would be exactly similar in both cases. Under such circumstances, all the muscles below the knee would become atrophied from the want of exercise, if nothing worse were experienced.

78. The above illustration, although an extreme one, shows the absurdity of a boot or shoe made of rigid material. If we propose to improve an organized body of so elastic, sensitive, and complicated a structure as the human foot, it must be by means adapted to its peculiar vitality, as has already been shown (63—68), and not as we shoe rocking levers, wooden legs, and the feet of horses and donkeys.

79. The requirements of the foot being different at different ages (48), these differences will now be very briefly noticed.

80. In infancy we have seen (48) that the foot is broad at the toes and narrow at the tarsus—that the bones are soft, and the whole of the parts in a tender state. At this period the foot is growing rapidly, and, like all other organized bodies under similar circumstances, it is easily injured by external pressure; but when suitable provision is made for its natural wants and protection, internally and externally, it arrives at maturity free from deformity—

all its parts being fully developed, and in a healthy state.

81. Exercise we have also seen (68) is essential to health and the growth of muscle, tendon, ligament, and bone ; and this is just what all healthy children delight in, viz. exercise by all sorts of sprawling and jumping, and what they should daily have—plenty of running about in the open air, their legs and feet being exposed as much as possible to the stimulating influence of light ; the foot being in the free enjoyment of all its functions, *i. e.* every toe and articulation having free play.

82. A proper covering for the foot in childhood is thus a very important question, as upon it depends the free action of all its parts, so essential to health and strength (68, 69), and without which exercise cannot be taken with advantage (70). It is so at every period of life, but doubly so at this tender age, because of the soft state of the muscles, tendons, ligaments, and bones (48, 80), and the fact that the foot is growing and daily increasing in size.

83. The shoemaker, then, has not only to make provision for the wide outspread toes of a child, the narrow and soft tarsal bones, the concavity of the inside of the foot (80), and the general elasticity and mobility of parts (76), but for the growing length, breadth, and increasing dimensions of the whole extremities.

84. I have been the more anxious to impress

these facts upon the attention of my readers, because when I come to examine in a subsequent section (162), how far the stockings and shoes now made for children meet the requirements of their feet—the general rule carried out will be found the very reverse of the provisions just noticed—the shoe being narrow in front instead of broad—to afford room for the breadth of the toes; convex at the inside instead of concave, to provide for the concavity of the inside of the foot; rigid at the waist, instead of elastic, to provide for the elasticity of the instep under pressure, and the backward elongation of the foot in walking; and pinching the foot everywhere, instead of possessing suitable provision for the healthy development of its delicate structure and beautiful mechanism (219). With such an anomalous state of things before me daily, they will, I trust, appreciate the earnestness with which I advocate inquiry into the peculiar wants of the foot in childhood—a period when the feet of the helpless and innocent creatures are but too frequently crammed into pinching shoes, by unthinking mothers and angry, unfeeling nurses.

85. After three or four years' exercise in running about, the foot of the child begins to exhibit greater firmness in the handling under measurement for a shoe; and from this period onwards to twelve and fourteen years of age, the feet of boys and girls require great attention in the shoeing, to preserve

them in their normal form and beauty, owing to the little care which they themselves take of their feet, and the rough treatment they sometimes experience in driving amongst each other at school. It is very remarkable indeed, to contemplate what boys' feet will endure when running about barefoot, and not a little humiliating to think that the barefooted urchins who run about the streets of London have healthier and better-formed feet than those of the many princely juvenile establishments, where no expense is spared in stockings, boots, and shoes! The fact points to the very heavy responsibility under which parents' and guardians lie, relative to the peculiar requirements of a boy's foot at this age. No doubt it is not an easy matter to keep boys properly shod, so furiously do they drive against everything that stands in the way of their feet—every loose stone in the road getting a toss as they pass; but much better make them go barefoot than spoil their feet. In other respects, the foot at this age maintains all the characteristics of that of childhood, already noticed (83), for which provision must accordingly be made.

86. From the age of fourteen to twenty years, the foot gradually assumes a more matured form, the tarsus becoming thicker—a characteristic that gives to the toes proportionally a narrower appearance. By this time, too, young people begin to think for themselves, and to be guided too often more by mistaken

notions of fashion than the comfort of their feet. The consequence of this is soon told, for they bring upon themselves, throughout the after-period of life, the very thing they wish to avoid—*ill-shapen feet;* while along with distorted toes and an ungraceful mode of walking, they experience, often long before old age overtakes them, an amount of suffering from corns, bunions, and inflamed joints, that is wholly indescribable. During the greater part of this period, if not the whole, the foot is still growing, so that provision has to be made in the size of the covering for this increase ;—to do so, new boots, shoes, and stockings require to be made as large as possible, so that the former shall not shuffle on the feet, and the latter form into folds. They should all be light, so as not to encumber growing muscles with unnecessary weight, and should be constructed of elastic material; and they should regularly be thrown aside whenever they begin to pinch the toes, so as to turn them from their normal position, deforming the feet.

87. This, too, is that particular period of life when parents and guardians are relieved of much, if not all, responsibility as to dress. It, therefore, becomes young people, in taking this responsibility upon themselves, to study practically the normal form of their feet, and to cultivate their health and strength by regular exercise, making themselves thoroughly acquainted with their beautiful me-

chanism, and the elastic movements of their several parts, so essentially necessary to the gracefulness and dignity of an easy, health-giving step in walking. It is not my duty or interest to say a word against fashion, but fashion ought to add usefulness and beauty to the appearance of the boot or shoe, without producing deformity of structure to the foot, and its consequent—a limping unsightliness of gait in walking. That which gives rise to the latter cannot by any legitimate means produce the former, for beauty and deformity are incompatible terms. Because fashion proposes broad-toed shoes to-day, round ones to-morrow, and narrow the next day, that is no reason for young people interfering with the external anatomy and healthy mechanical functions of their feet; for it is just as necessary to be particular about the geographical position of one's toes, as about that of the counties of a kingdom, or the empires of the world; and when young people begin to shape their feet on the same principle that the blacksmith shapes a ploughshare on his anvil, there is obviously something radically wrong, or fundamentally wanting in their education.

88. Much of what has just been said of youth, in the last paragraph, is applicable to manhood and old age. The foot, although it has now attained to maturity, is still subject to all the changes peculiar to organic life, such as the daily waste, daily repairs, and any extra tear and wear from exercise; conse-

quently, provision has to be made in the shoeing for the free action of all the vital functions in these several respects. Indeed, one of the chief characteristics of manhood is the liability of the foot to injury from severe strains upon the muscles, under the many pedestrian feats to which it is, at this period, subject; and from the heavy burdens often borne, and the extra pressure so frequently and thoughtlessly laid upon the arch of the foot, exceeding the maximum elasticity and expansibility which it is capable of bearing. Provision, therefore, has to be made for such extremes, so as to afford man at this period of life every opportunity that can be embraced to cultivate health and strength, so as to avoid atrophy and its consequents. Again, corpulency, rigidity of structure, and muscular weakness are the common concomitants of old age; the foot becoming more and more tender after the meridian of life is passed—conditions that call for a very diversified provision as to the nature of the covering.

89. Clerks, and all engaged in sedentary occupations, are a class requiring, at every period of life, stockings to fit comfortably the feet, and light roomy boots or shoes, so as to allow a free circulation of the vital fluid, and to permit of the free action of the toes, instep, and ankles, a provision which will be found to afford great relief when confined close at the desk,—relief, too, which the foot naturally strives to obtain.

90. Merchants and others behind the counter are another class whose feet require special provision. Although they have more free exercise than those of clerks, yet continuous standing is trying for the feet, especially of young people; ample provision should therefore be made for them accordingly, by an easy elastic covering to expand freely under the pressure of the foot, which has sometimes to sustain heavy weights in lifting packages and other goods. It can never be too closely borne in mind that *it is from extremes that the foot suffers harm;* and that it is for such extremes, therefore, that provision ought to be made in the shoeing.

91. Millers, coal-porters, carriers, hawkers, house-carpenters, masons, and the building trades generally, form another class demanding special attention. They require stronger boots and shoes than either of the previous examples, because they are more exposed to the weather. In this case, the feet have generally plenty of exercise daily to keep them in health, if they are allowed free action in the boot or shoe worn. They have heavy burdens occasionally to carry—often up or down inclined gangways, stairs, ladders, and slanting roofs of houses, so that the muscles of the feet and legs should be increased in strength for the same (68).

92. Farmers, ploughmen, shepherds, and others engaged in husbandry, as also sportsmen, tourists, &c., are much exposed to the weather—to walking

amongst grass, clods, stones, and the like; consequently they require boots and shoes suitable for their peculiar occupations. The foot in this case is often subject to very severe exercise, both in walking and in carrying heavy burdens, and therefore the cultivation of its health and strength by the free action of all the muscles (68) is imperatively necessary.

93. Soldiers may be taken as another class requiring special notice. In modern tactics, an army boot or shoe has become a proposition of so much importance, that I have thought it absolutely necessary to devote to it a special chapter (IX.), and to which I here refer for detail. This arises from a threefold cause—Improvements in military science;* the necessity of improving the physical condition of the soldier;† and the climate of India, in which

* "War in modern times consists so much in the science of making men march, for the purpose of striking an unexpected blow on the enemy, that the efficiency of soldiers depends greatly on their capacity for executing long marches with comparative ease. Marshal Saxe and General Foy, both of whom had great military experience, do not hesitate in stating that the secret of war lies in the power of marching—namely, in the strength of the legs."—*Henry Marshall, Dep. Insp. Gen. of Hospitals, on Enlistment,* 1839.

† Marshal Saxe, in his Memoirs, says:—"In regard to the legs and feet, I could wish the soldiers were to have shoes made of thin leather, with low heels, which will fit extremely well, and make them involuntarily assume a good grace in marching; because low heels oblige men to turn out their toes, to stretch their joints, and consequently draw in their shoulders."

the British soldier has such important duties to perform.*

94. Sailors and all seafaring people form another special class, the health and muscular strength of whose feet require cultivation, and whose shoes, therefore, should be light, easy, elastic ones, fitting well and closely to the feet.

95. Again, the foot requires lighter shoes in summer than in winter, in southern latitudes than in northern ones, for reasons too obvious to require mention.

* A distinguished writer on Indian affairs thus expresses himself:—"We are almost led to wish to see the European soldier similarly prepared for his toilsome march, unencumbered by the unyielding shoe, which sometimes becomes in the day a source of greater annoyance than comfort to him ; he would be enabled to undertake fatigue and privations for which he is now totally unprepared; he would find an elastic tread, a firm command over his muscular system follow upon such a plan ; he would be capable of making a charge upon the enemy with greater steadiness, and enabled to bear the shock which he is now less capable of resisting. In this respect we should do well to imitate the native soldier of India, who, under the English banner, has followed Clive, Hastings, or Keane, when the British soldier has almost sunk from the insuperable difficulties which attend wearing all parts of the dress he has been accustomed to do in England, forgetful of the climate in which he is placed."

## CHAPTER V.

### ON THE MEASUREMENT OF THE FOOT.—ON THE STOCKING AND LAST.

96. In the preceding chapters, frequent allusion has been made to the ever-varying form of the foot, and its consequent diversity of measurement and other circumstances, for which provision has to be made in the shoeing of man. In this chapter, the measurement of the foot, the form and construction of the stocking, and the character of the last will be discussed, with a view to their application in the cutting and fitting department.

97. The following diagram illustrates the usual mode of measurement, in a manner that requires no explanation to those who have been measured. The length of the foot is first taken by a rule when in repose; then the different girths, as shown by the figures 2 to 7; and lastly, the foot is placed flat upon a page of an outline book, or atlas of the sole, when the

outline is traced with a pencil, the person standing upon the foot being measured, so as to show its elongation,—the outline thus giving both the length and breadth of the foot under pressure.

98. The difference between the length of the measurement of the foot taken in repose and that of the outline in the atlas shows the amount of elongation of the foot under the simple pressure of the weight of the body (27), when the heel and toes recede from each other like the ends of the spring of a carriage under the weight of a load, and which is very different under different circumstances.

99. In this elongation of the sole provision should always be made for extremes (28), so as to prevent the foot sustaining injury, when extra pressure is borne by the arch, as in jumping and carrying heavy burdens down stairs, and the like. In some occupations we have seen the foot is more subject to extreme pressure of this kind than in others (40); while some feet are more easily flattened from muscular weakness than others; but all feet experience less or more of it, in extreme cases, so that, unless provision is made for the greatest expansion under such circumstances, the foot must inevitably sustain injury. And it is but proper to remark that the less the foot is accustomed to such extremes the more likely is it to receive harm. In some finely-arched long feet, having strong powerful muscles, tendons, and ligaments, the elongation under the

mere weight of the body in the measuring is often very little, and yet when such feet are subjected to a sudden jerk or pressure, especially if under a languid state of the muscles, the flattening of the arch is considerable, and the liability to danger great in a corresponding degree, from the consequent elongation of the foot, which in several instances that have come under my experience, has measured fully one inch more under pressure than when in repose.

100. As this elongation takes place at the instep, or between the piers of the arch—the piers, or heel, and anterior part of the metatarsus receding from each other, provision should consequently be made in the waist of the boot or shoe for this elongation. The heel and toes of the nude foot in travelling slip or recede from each other upon the ground; but the heel and toe of the stocking, from being always less or more moist with perspiration, especially in extremes of exercise in warm weather, will not slip—and even if under force they did so, the friction would be intolerable, consequently elongation at the heel and toe of the boot or shoe is incompatible with the circumstances of the case. It is, therefore, at the waist, and waist alone, that the boot or shoe must expand to meet the elongation of the corresponding part of the foot; and it will readily be seen, that in the measurement of the foot for its covering, special attention requires to be paid to the peculiar charac-

## MEASUREMENT OF THE FOOT.

teristics of its anatomical structure, so as to provide for extremes (23, 76, 99).

101. In the growing foot, however, provision requires to be made at the toe of the boot or shoe for the foot's increasing length and expansibility; and as these are often very irregular as to amount, sometimes growing fast, sometimes slow, no little judgment is required on the part of the shoemaker, to make suitable provision for all the circumstances involved, especially in examples of delicate health, or of temperaments subject to inflammatory attacks, as in them the slightest pressure in the extreme of heat or cold is certain to produce harm of some kind or other.

102. Again, in measuring the length of the foot, provision requires to be made for the second kind of elongation (29)—that which takes place forwards when the toes are bent upwards (30), and that which takes place backwards when the heel rises from the ground (31).

103. If the waist of the boot or shoe is made of sufficiently elastic material, it will stretch so as to make provision for the latter elongation backwards (31); but for the elongation in front (30) the boot or shoe will require to be made longer at the toe than the foot, and the extra length will depend upon the peculiar characteristics of the bend of the foot at the metatarsal articulations with the toes.

104. It will thus be seen, that in measuring the

length of the foot, the shoemaker has to place more dependance upon his skill and judgment in the matter, than upon what the rule and atlas indicate. Any workman can take the length of the foot with a rule, and trace its outline on a slip of paper; but a knowledge of its anatomical structure is absolutely necessary, as Dr. Camper justly observes, to enable any one to make the necessary provision for extremes, both in the growing and full-grown foot, to which attention has just been drawn.

105. Having taken the length of the foot, we next come to consider what provision is necessary for the toes, whose external anatomy was examined, from 41 to 48, to which the reader is referred. The depth or thickness of the great toe at the point (43) is shown in the diagram, 97, at 1, and the girth, breadth, and thickness at the bend or tread of the foot (46 and 47) is shown at 2. The outline upon the atlas is also necessary to determine the breadth of the foot, the length of the toes, and the angular form of the foot in front, and bend at the metatarsal hinge (44 and 45).

106. The proper measurement of this part of the foot, including the toes and metatarsus, is a most important affair. This arises from the peculiar multiplicity of bones and articulations in its mechanism, and from the dependance of the general health of the foot, and even of the whole body upon the free action of every bone, tendon, ligament, and

muscle of which it is formed. This has been shown in the last chapter, more especially under sections 59, 69, and 72, to which the reader is referred. Indeed, the pinching of the toes has proverbially a significant meaning as regards the sanitary condition of the foot and general health of the body.

107. The girth around the toes at 2 (97), where they articulate with the metatarsus, although usually relied upon, is nevertheless far from an adequate measurement of this part of the foot. Indeed, it were difficult to conceive anything more unsatisfactory than it is, for even with the atlas and the outline which it gives of the breadth and angular form in front, much remains undetermined by either girth or outline that has to be supplied by the judgment of the shoemaker. The truth of this is very forcibly illustrated by transverse sections of the casts of feet of different forms, girths, and breadths at 2 in the diagram. In examples of this kind, it will be found that girthing the foot here is something analogous to a joiner girthing a tenon of an irregular, circular, or polygonal form, in order to make a mortise for it. It is not more the duty of the joiner to attend to the peculiar shape of his tenon, so as to make for it a mortise to fit in every respect, than it is the duty of the shoemaker to attend to the peculiar forms of transverse sections of the human foot, in order to provide a proper covering for it.

108. The main points for which special provision

has to be made, are the breadth across the tread at 2, the length between 1 and 2, the extra length in the toe of the boot or shoe, required to allow the toes to bend upwards, and the exact curvature and thickness of the edge of the foot round the toes from the line 2 on the inside, to the same line on the outside, or from the root of the great toe on the inside to the root of the little toe on the outside. The former three are more easily determined than the latter one. Indeed, if provision is made for the thickness and curvature of the edge of the foot, the three first questions will be solved.

109. The two outside toes, it will thus be observed, demand special protection, as upon their welfare that of the others between mainly depend. It is therefore necessary, in compliance with this demand, that the exact measurement of the thickness of the great toe and the thickness of the little toe, including the peculiar position and curvature of each on the outside, for which provision has to be made, should be attended to; for without this, it is impossible to preserve them in their normal position, and to prevent them from injuriously interfering with the freedom of those between, less able naturally to defend themselves. This is necessary, not only to allow all the toes being kept in their proper position, but also to secure for them their free action, at the same time, for the purpose of cultivating their health and strength (68), and thus

qualifying them for whatever duties they have to perform.

110. Referring again to the diagram (97), the other girths, 3, 4, 5, and 6, are, for similar reasons, equally inadequate to secure the proper measurement of the metatarsus and tarsus—or of the instep, heel, and ankle—"a proper fit" depending less upon their accuracy as to superficial length, than upon the judgment of the shoemaker as to their respective contents. In illustration of this, readers may be referred to what has already been said on the external anatomy of these parts severally in a former chapter (sections 51 to 57). In taking each of these girths, the shoemaker has to attend to the peculiar configuration of the part, and the outline which a transverse section of it would present to his eye, as if such were actually taken, and also to the outline which a longitudinal section of the foot (page 46) and leg would present, similar to the outline of what is shown in the diagram, before he can set to work successfully at the cutting-bench in the application of his measurement, so as to get the different parts of the boot or shoe to fit the corresponding parts of the foot ; as, for example, the external points 1, 2, 3, 4, 5, 6 of the foot to fit the corresponding internal parts of the boot, and so on, for the different points of the sole and heel.

111. We next come to the heel, a division or portion of the foot that receives less attention,

generally, in the measurement than it merits. If it is the strongest part, it is because it has the most work to do, and therefore there is the greater need to make the necessary provision for enabling it to discharge its functions. When we come to examine how far demands of this kind are complied with in the thick rigid soles and high heels so fashionable among certain classes (Chaps. VIII. and IX.), it will be found that the normal functions of this important part of the foot are sacrificed, and along with them almost all the functions of the other parts already noticed, *i.e.* the instep and toes. This arises from the important leverage the heel, with the tendons and muscles attached to it, plays in the peculiar functions it has to perform, and for which special provision has consequently to be made in the measurement. We have seen, for example, the compensation in part (32) of the backward elongation of the foot by the downward bending of the heel, as when a person stands in the tip-toe attitude, or as in going up or down stairs—up or down a steep incline, &c. In this position, the metatarsus or instep is brought nearly into a line with the leg, so that the calf of the leg on the one side of the heel-bone, and the lenticular bone or tread of the foot on the other side, are both brought nearer to the heel by the amount of contraction of the muscles of the calf of the leg and of the sole of the foot, consequently the span of the foot is shortened, and the arch of necessity raised. Now, to comply with this peculiar function of the heel and its tackle, the waist of the boot or shoe must bend inwards, and the heel downwards, in harmony with the respective movements of the corresponding parts of the foot. These are conditions imperatively demanded, and special attention requires to be drawn to them. They are very different in different feet; but in each case special provision has to be made in the measurement of the waist, heel, and corresponding parts of the uppers, as will be shown in a subsequent chapter (VII.) on the cutting department.

112. In the measurement of the foot, another topic that claims special attention is the manner many "go over the sole," sometimes to the inside, but perhaps more frequently to the outside. This is a source of great inconvenience, often accompanied with no little pain to those who wear their shoes in this manner. The root of the evil may arise from a defect in the manufacture of the boot or shoe worn at the time; but not unfrequently from a deformity in the form of the leg or foot, or both. Children often experience great weakness about the feet, ankles, and knees, requiring very great care to get them to grow right, so as to walk fairly on the sole. Indeed, all children require great attention in this respect; and when neglected, the line of gravitation will be found either on the one side or the other, as

the case may be, of the centre of the heel, and for this divergence special provision requires to be made in the manufacture of the boot or shoe,—sometimes one way, sometimes another,—just as the peculiar circumstances of the case may direct.

113. Both feet should be measured to ascertain if they are alike. In appearance it may be impossible to distinguish any difference; but it not unfrequently occurs that there is a considerable diversity in the measurement, after all, even in the case of sound, healthy feet. And, what is more, feet at one time of life may be alike, and yet different at another; while the feet of many old people, who have been subject to sedentary habits, are liable to swell by night, often not equally, and for every diversity of this kind the requisite provision should be made.

114. The length, breadth, thickness, position, and edge curvature of the toes; the different girths, and distances between them; the peculiarities of the arch of the instep, and of the projection of the heel; the heights of the different points 2, 3, 4, 5, and 6 in the diagram (97), above the base-line or sole, 1, on which the foot rests; and the outlines which transverse and longitudinal sections of casts would present to the eye of the workman taking their measurement, must all be carefully noted for subsequent application in the cutting department, as we have thus endeavoured to show.

115. How does the stocking make provision for the different conditions thus briefly reviewed in the last section (114)? To this the practical answer of the vast majority of cases that daily come under the notice of the shoemaker is far from favourable to the inner covering, as now generally worn, for in ninety-nine cases perhaps out of every hundred the source of injury to the toes is in the toe of the stocking.

116. The period at which the injury referred to above commences is childhood, when the foot is growing, the parts tender, and the toes spreading (80—84). At this helpless period of life the delicately-feeble, outspreading toes are wedged into a narrow-toed stocking, often so short as to double in the toes, diminishing the length of the rapidly-growing foot! It is next, perhaps, tightly laced into a boot of less interior dimensions than itself; when the poor little creature is left to sprawl about, with a limping, stumping gait, thus learning to walk as it best can under circumstances the most cruel and torturing imaginable. Such examples are too frequently characterized by a degree of indifference to the welfare of growing feet that merits a worse designation than I shall give it,—thoughtless mothers and guardians neglecting their charge in a manner that calls loudly for public interference and exposure, in order, if possible, to remedy such *an unnatural state of things*. Often, too, where the stocking is

sufficiently large—or, it may be, *over-large*—it narrows to a point in front, into which the tender spreading toes of the child are wedged by the act of forcing its foot into the boot, the loose stocking at the heel only serving to make matters worse by wedging the metatarsus and toes forward into the narrow-toed stocking and boot. Were it a garden vegetable—as a turnip, potato, carrot, cucumber, or any other growing organism, save the foot of an innocent child, no pains would be spared to cultivate its healthy development! but the foot of the child at this tender age, how often is it injured by the stocking! And when the work of malformation is once begun, it seldom finishes with childhood, or even youth and manhood, but gradually progresses from bad to worse, bringing upon old age a state of suffering too often wholly attributed to the outer covering.

117. Ought not the stocking to have toes, so to speak, like the foot? The question is put purposely to afford every freedom of inquiry and discussion merited. Stockings are now being manufactured with toes, and pretty extensively worn, and there cannot be a doubt but they have many qualities to recommend them to general use amongst all classes of society; for were the growing toes to enjoy unrestrained liberty of action in such a covering, they would then be found presenting the beautifully-proportioned symmetry of the fingers of the hand. Why should the toes be

atrophied and deformed as they now so commonly are, if means so simple are capable of promoting their healthy development? When growing toes are squeezed together in a shapeless knot, as it were, they become so atrophied as to lose, not only their muscular strength, but their normal individuality, so to speak, whilst they are infinitely more subject to gout and all sorts of disease, than when kept separate in the full enjoyment of their functions in a toed stocking, and in a properly constructed boot or shoe. No doubt toes thus squeezed and atrophied, when first put into such a covering, would feel, as it were, from home; but those who have some experience in the matter, affirm that they soon begin to recover health, strength, and symmetry from the stimulating action of the stocking on the functions of the delicately fine skin between the toes and the formation of healthy tissue, every toe gradually developing its natural beauty and individuality. When the ALL-WISE CREATOR designed the foot of man, toes were given for a wise purpose, and a similar award may one day be pronounced in favour of toes to stockings.

118. The foot in a stocking with toes requires a broader boot or shoe in front, but in other respects is rather more easily measured and fitted in the shoeing than when the common stocking is worn. This arises from the toes being always less or more squeezed into the latter, so that their normal dimensions are more difficult to be obtained with accuracy;

whereas, when the former is worn, configuration is more easily seen.

119. The next topic for consideration is the Last. Its measurement must correspond with the requirements of the foot. It has been shown (41—57) that feet differ in form in such a manner as to admit of classification; and in a similar manner I classify lasts, so that I know at once where to find the peculiar shape required on obtaining the measurement of a customer's foot.

120. With the regular customer whose boot or shoe, according to the kind, such as a dress-boot, &c. &c., is always made upon the same last, there is little difficulty experienced in applying the measurement, as the two are booked together, and hence are directly found each under its respective number in its own class.

121. With an order for the first time, it is often otherwise, as a last corresponding to the measurement has to be provided.

122. Every customer, however, should have his or her own last for every size of boot or shoe intended to be worn. It may, therefore, be set down as a rule, that every foot ought to have its own last; and simple as such a rule may appear at first sight to be, and to some perhaps superfluous, no one who wishes a proper fit should lose sight of its real value in practice.

123. As the last-maker seldom or never sees the

foot for which he has to make a last, it is no easy matter communicating to him what has been said in the preceding part of this chapter relative to measurement. As the foot is the pattern for which the last has to be made, perhaps the simplest and surest plan to secure a proper fit is a cast of the foot for his guidance, as, with a proper cast before him, and an easy-fitting old boot or shoe, as the case may be, to try the last, he will be able to make the necessary difference between the cast and the last, that the circumstances of the case require. But whichever plan is adopted, the last should be a proper fit; and every one who can afford it should have his own boot-trees at home, to preserve his boots in their proper shape, and, what is not undeserving of attention, to permit of their being cleaned more easily and better than they can be otherwise.

## CHAPTER VI.

### ON RAW MATERIALS, HIDES, LEATHER, ETC.

124. THE materials of which boots and shoes are generally constructed, do not appear to be very well adapted for the purpose. Indeed, it requires no practical evidence to show that they are deficient in many respects, affording in bad weather a very imperfect protection to the foot, while they do not preserve it in that uniform degree of temperature which the extremes of our climate demand. They, in short, do not make suitable provision for the physical well-being of the foot. There is however, at present, a very strong current of inquiry in favour of improvement; and as the field is wide and promising, I shall do little more in this chapter than take a very cursory glance at the subject, confining my remarks chiefly to those topics more especially requiring discussion, taking it for granted that my readers are aware that the manufacture of the various materials in question are pretty fully treated in the different encyclopædias, and similar works comprising the popular literature of the day.

125. The great bulk of the boots and shoes worn in this country is now, as it has been from time immemorial, manufactured of leather procured from the

skins of the domesticated animals that supply us with labour and butcher-meat. Leadenhall Market furnishes an interesting example of what the butchers of the British capital alone supply weekly. In addition to the home supply, a large number of foreign hides are also required to supply the home demand.

126. Early maturity and the extra fattening of stock by farmers, on the one hand, coupled with the more rapid processes of manufacture on the other, from improvements in the chemical agents employed, are all exercising certain influences upon the quality of leather, and the common complaint is, that the quality, upon the whole, is not improving.

127. There cannot be a doubt that " the rage for cheap boots and shoes " has given rise to the splitting of hides and rapid processes for producing an inferior article. This is but the common course of things, and it would be unreasonable to suppose an article like leather an exception to this rule. But the more intelligent of the public are now beginning to experience the short-sighted economy of cheap leather, the higher-priced article proving itself the cheapest in the end.

128. To notice or even enumerate the various kinds of tanned, curried, and tawed leathers used by shoemakers would be superfluous, as all must be familiar with them. In a country like this, there must of necessity be variety in its most comprehen-

sive sense, to supply the different demands of so many occupations and ranks of society.

129. The principal objections to leather as generally manufactured at present is, that a hide, however well tanned it may be, is not of uniform quality throughout; that, irrespective of this difference of quality, no little difficulty is experienced in laying in stock, where the hides are in other respects equal to each other, from the various injuries they sustain before the animal is slaughtered—such as when the skin is kept continually wet and in an unhealthy state, from inattention to cleanliness in fattening. Again, that, when made into boots and shoes, leather, both soles and uppers, is liable to become rigid and hard, and that even when kept pliant and flexible it is non-elastic, and therefore unsuited to the contractility and expansibility of the foot; while when wet is kept out by means of grease and other repellants, the perspiration of the foot is at the same time kept in, to the injury of health.

130. It is rather singular that an article, subject to so many heavy objections, should be so extensively and almost exclusively used to this day as a covering for the foot of man, when the world presents so many other articles used in the manufacture of dress. In the primitive state of society the skins of animals had, no doubt, many things to recommend them; but the progress of civilization and of science is evidently going ahead of the leathers now in use, and so fast,

that the present state of things, generally speaking, is manifestly out of date; while the improvements in the mechanical characteristics of boots and shoes being introduced, together with the elastic articles of which they are manufactured, form the commencement of a new era in shoemaking.

131. Of late years various manufactures have been introduced for the purpose of obviating objections of the above nature, and effecting the improvements contemplated. It is now about twenty-five years since I introduced elasticated leather into the soles of boots and shoes, and certain parts of the uppers; prior to 1835, I had tried caoutchouc in various ways; and at the present moment there is a strong bent of inclination in favour of different kinds of manufactured fabrics both for soles and uppers, although nothing deserving of special notice has yet been discovered and sufficiently tested at the bar of experience, to be received as a standard substitute for leather. At the same time, substantial progress is annually being made in this direction. Those who advocate the exclusive use of leather, must admit the increasing demand for manufactures of an elastic quality, including improvements in the manufacture of animal skin itself.

132. Principles always merit the attention of practical men, and there are two principles involved in carrying out the above movement deserving of notice. In the first of these, the manufactured

fabrics in question are only used in part, as gutta-percha soles, elasticated leather waists, sides or gores, fronts, &c., the principal portion of the boot or shoe being made, as usual, of leather. In the other case a thinner boot or shoe, wholly made of leather, or partly so, as in the first case, is worn in fine weather, and over it an *over-shoe* of elasticated material in wet weather. Both have special claims upon attention.

133. In this twofold line of operation the reader cannot fail to perceive a practical acknowledgment of the above objections embodied, and also at the same time a spirit of progress at work that will one day unquestionably triumph over all opposition in the way of a perfect covering for the foot, however dark may be the clouds that surround the problem at present.

## CHAPTER VII.

### ON THE CONSTRUCTION OF BOOTS AND SHOES.

134. In this chapter the work in the cutting and manufacturing departments of the trade will briefly be reviewed. In both branches the principal amount of the work must be learned by serving an apprenticeship, and not by reading books; and therefore our observations will be confined to those principles involved in applying the measurements of a former chapter—in cutting them out, and in putting them upon the last. We shall also very briefly notice those principles involved in the ebbing and flowing tide of fashion.

135. In applying the measurements, the first thing, of course, demanding attention is the kind of boot or shoe ordered. Is it, for example, a Wellington? a Blucher? an Albert? an elastic side? a lacing shoe? or what? But into details of this kind it will be unnecessary to enter. In each case the foot has its peculiar demands, as stated in the measurement (114), and it is with conditions of this kind that we have almost exclusively to deal.

136. In cutting out of a hide the several parts that are to form a boot or shoe, we find there is a wide

difference between the back, flank, and belly, as to quality, whether it is prepared for sole or upper, that calls for the special exercise of no little judgment before the knife is entered, in order to economize the whole, and yet do justice to all parties. Of late this has become, as it were, a special branch of the trade by itself, the several parts being in some cases cut by machinery, but more generally yet by the hand, so that if wished they can now be had separately, of any quality and quantity.

137. It is only, however, when the shoemaker begins to finish the several parts of the "uppers" for "*sewing*" and "*lasting*," that his professional skill is called into requisition. Were the foot a cube—or any regular-sided body—St. Crispin's problem at the cutting-board would be easily solved ; but to fit the toes, the instep, the ankle, and the heel (114), is a very different affair—a work that requires an apprenticeship of several years to learn it, as already stated ; and when this is done, only but a few journeymen are ever fairly masters of it. Any attempt to make it intelligible on paper would inevitably prove abortive. If properly done, the cutting is a fine piece of workmanship, and those who have a talent for it are valuable servants in a large establishment.

138. Much professional skill is also required in putting the uppers properly upon the last, so that every part shall occupy its proper place. Unless

this is carefully attended to, some parts, as at the great toe, will be over-stretched, while others will be the reverse, so that the boot or shoe, after it begins to be worn, will lose its proper shape, in consequence of the leather returning to its original unstretched dimensions.

139. In every case the uppers have to undergo a certain amount of stretching at the toes, the instep, ankle, and around the edge of the last, at the sole, so that the successful performance of the work depends upon each part being just stretched as it ought to be, neither less nor more. This will readily be understood by attending to the configuration of one's own boot, and reflecting for a moment that the several parts of which it is made are cut from a plain superficies or even piece of leather. It will also be understood why new boots or shoes are so liable to get out of shape, especially in wet weather, and why boot-trees are of so much service.

140. The peculiar thickness and shape of the sole are topics that have engrossed considerable diversity of opinion, both as to style and durability. As to the former, much of the general appearance of the boot or shoe depends upon the thickness and configuration of the sole, and, accordingly, it is one of those parts that is more than ordinarily subject to the caprice of fashion.

141. A thin flexible sole, of good material, will last longer in proportion to its thickness than a

thick, rigid, and hard one. This arises from the ease with which the former is worn. The foot, for example, from possessing its mechanical freedom, walks lighter, or more naturally and softly on the ground, on the one hand, and from the extra friction, tear and wear, to which the latter is subject, on the other hand, all the movements of the sole being of a hammering destructive character on the ground. Hence, the reason why large hobnails are so soon worn in the thick-soled lacing-boot of our agricultural labourers, draymen, waggoners, &c. &c. Without travelling into details, the conclusion is manifest, that thick rigid soles are a false economy, in a two-fold sense, to those who wear them.

142. With regard to shape, the sole of the boot or shoe should in principle bear a close relationship to that of the foot or its outline upon the atlas (97, 105). How far it may be legitimately interfered with by fashion, will be noticed in a subsequent section (151). The sole is the bearing on which the piers of the foot or the heel and anterior part of the metatarsus rest, and therefore should harmonize with their movements; consequently it must elongate under pressure (99), bending upwards at the waist, and downwards at the heel, as formerly shown (111).

143. The sole, it will thus be seen, with the necessary elongation required cannot be cut out of the ordinary sole leather, either in one piece or other-

wise, but must have elastic material that will elongate and bend easily at the waist, somehow or other, introduced. Of the elasticated material introduced by myself long ago, I shall treat afterwards (Chap. X.). At present, I am discussing a principle necessary to be attended to in reference to the character of the sole of the boot or shoe to harmonize with a corresponding characteristic of the foot.

144. In walking, only a small part of the sole of the nude foot touches the ground. A print of the wet foot on the floor affords a practical illustration of this fact. The form of this print will be found very different in different feet. In some, comparatively flat or very low-arched ones, the whole of the outside, from the little toe to the heel, touches the ground, so that the outline of the print, in such cases, forms an irregularly-shaped figure, the bearings of the two piers of the longitudinal arch being connected by a long narrow bearing on the outside, under what may be termed the pier of the lateral arch (33 and 49—53).

145. Between the form or outline of this print or bearing of the nude foot upon the ground and the shape of the sole of the boot or shoe, there ought always to be a more close relationship than even between it and the outline upon the atlas, already noticed.

146. In common phraseology this peculiarity in the shape of the sole is known by the technical

expression of "right" and "left," first used to distinguish a pair of boots or shoes thus made on two lasts, one for each foot—a right and a left—from a pair made on one last, and worn alternately on both feet.

147. This curving or hollowing out of the sole on the inside is absolutely necessary for the special purpose of permitting the instep to be properly clothed on the under-side. The best illustration of this will be found in the examination of this part of one's own boot or shoe, as that cannot fail to carry conviction to the mind that, if the sole were equally straight on both sides, the under-side of the instep would not fit close and well to the foot.

148. The clothing of the under-side of the instep, as to extent, is different, both longitudinally and laterally in differently-arched feet, being greatest in those having a high broad arch, and least in those having a low narrow one; consequently the concavity of the inner side of the sole ought to correspond therewith, and therefore should be greatest in the former examples and least in the latter.

149. In the manufacture of ready-made boots and shoes machinery has of late years been making progress, being now largely used in the sewing of much of the plain work of the uppers. This movement is also increasing the trade in ready-made uppers for a certain class of customer-work.

150. Soles are generally sewed to the uppers on

the old plan, too well known to require notice. The riveting system, long ago introduced by Brunel, sen., has recently been reintroduced with some improvements; but the plan may not inaptly be said to be as yet devoid of that degree of merit deserving a more detailed notice, or of demerit calling for exposure.

151. With regard to Fashion, she has acquired no legitimate right to interfere injuriously with the normal form and physical well-being of the human foot. In other respects it would be unwise to set very narrow and illiberal limits to the boundary of her province.

152. There is, however, one peculiar view of this subject that cannot be passed over so smoothly; namely, fallacious, empirical notions relative to the shape and form of the boot or shoe, that are incompatible with the natural beauty of the human foot. In a former section (87) some plain hints to youth were thrown out, that render it unnecessary to say more here than merely express a regret that savage tribes should have a more correct and dignified conception of the foot of man than civilized nations! The fact is certainly a humbling one when viewed in its proper light, as we shall see when we come to examine fashionable boots and shoes, with their deforming results. At present, we shall only further observe that books have been written by very eminent men, well versed in physio-

logical science, on the pernicious effects of tight lacing on the spine of woman ; and it is much to be desired that the pen of some able writer were at work on a kindred subject,—the deformed feet of all civilized nations that wear fashionable boots and shoes ! Moreover, when in all our veterinary colleges professors are appointed to lecture on the best mode of shoeing our cattle, ought not professors to be appointed also at all our Universities to lecture on the best plan of shoeing mankind ?

## CHAPTER VIII.

ON THE CONSTRUCTION OF THE BOOTS AND SHOES NOW GENERALLY WORN, AND THEIR ADAPTATION TO THE FOOT.

153. In this chapter a few examples will be given to illustrate the present construction and general character of the boots and shoes commonly worn.

154. The strong lacing boot worn by agricultural labourers and a large class of hard-working people may be taken as the first example. When unlaced, it affords plenty of room to the foot, generally speaking, after it has arrived at maturity, being capacious at the heel and waist; but the moment it is laced the very reverse is experienced, the thick rigid leather closing upon the tarsus and metatarsus like a vice, and holding this part of the foot as rigidly fixed as if it were shod like a rocking lever, as formerly noticed (77 and 78). The rigid Bluchers and Wellingtons worn by another class (91) are little better.

155. The case of such a large portion of our industrial population demands a somewhat more detailed examination, for the twofold reason of ascertaining their present condition, and what they

require. In doing so, the observations made in this chapter will be confined to a general notice of the strong lacing boot of the agricultural labourer and others, reserving the principal amount of detail for the next chapter.

156. If the foot of an agricultural labourer is examined when his boot is tightly laced as above (154), the whole posterior part, including the heel, ankle, and instep, will be found so fixed into an angle formed by the rigid leather of the sole and uppers, as to destroy the mobility of this part of the foot. In point of fact, the shoeing of the human foot in rigid leather is thus similar in its effects to the shoeing of a rocking lever in cast iron (77). At the forepart it may bend a little, but the force required to do so takes an effort something analogous to that of jumping on one foot; so that under continuous exercise the muscles are soon exhausted. And what deserves special notice is the fact, that the muscles thus exhausted, as formerly shown (70), are not those whose natural function it is to bend the foot at the toes, but other muscles less able to perform the task, and hence more easily exhausted. The consequence of this is that the muscles of the heel, ankle, and instep, from comparative disuse, become so atrophied or wasted, that the labourer, when called upon to walk a long journey in a lighter boot, or more frequently a shoe, is so over-fatigued and "done up," to quote his own language, that he

often expresses a wish on the road for his heavy unbending boots, feeling satisfied, from daily experience, that in them he could accomplish the task more easily.

157. Examples of the above kind are of every-day occurrence, as when the poor workman on a Sunday or holiday visits his friends in his "Sunday shoes." They are cases of an extremely interesting character, especially when placed in contrast with those of the professional or trained pedestrian, accustomed to walk in light shoes; or even in contrast with Irishmen travelling to harvest, rope dancers, or other athletes, the health, strength, and muscular development of whose feet have been cultivated on sound philosophical principles, as formerly shown (68 to 73). Sir Charles Bell presents a very interesting contrast of this kind, pointing to the brawny leg of an Irish reaper in contrast with the "small and shapeless" leg of an English agricultural labourer, or those "whose feet and ankles are tightly laced in a shoe with a wooden sole."*

* Sir Charles Bell remarks, "That the whole apparatus of bones and joints being constituted in accurate relation to the muscular powers, it is preserved perfect by exercise; the tendons, the sheaths by which they are restrained, and the mucous bursus containing the lubricating fluid, can be seen in perfection only, when the animal machinery has been kept in *full activity.* In inflammation, and pain, and necessary restraint, they become weak; and even confinement and want of exercise, without disease, will produce imperfections. Exercise unfolds the mus-

158. The extra expenditure of muscular force in walking in strong laced boots must be considerable. We may be remiss in estimating results of this kind, but that does not reduce their value, or justify our want of duty and attention to facts thus exemplified. Even if we never for a moment once thought of the economy of muscle, on the one side, or its extravagant expenditure on the other, as exemplified in the case of the professional pedestrian walking in light easy shoes, and that of the agricultural labourer walking in his strong laced boots; a very great difference, nevertheless, exists, and its importance cannot be denied, for each example is in itself a faithful exposition of invaluable practical truth in this department of applied science.

159. The labourer walks with a jolting gait, like a man on stilts (as Sir Charles Bell very justly ob-

cular system, producing a full bold outline of the limbs, at the same time that the joints are knit small and clean. Look at the legs of a poor Irishman travelling to the harvest with bare feet; the thickness and roundness of the calf show that the foot and toes are free to permit the exercise of the muscles of the legs. Look again at the leg of our English peasant, whose foot and ankle are tightly laced in a shoe with a wooden sole, and you will perceive from the manner in which he lifts his legs, that the play of the ankle, foot, and toes, is lost, as much as if he went on stilts, and therefore are his legs small and shapeless: in short, the natural exercise of the parts, whether they be active or passive, is the stimulus to the circulation through them, exercise being as necessary to the perfect constitution of a bone as it is to the perfection of the muscular power."

serves), the movements in both cases being similar in principle. If in this example we assume, what few will deny, that it is better to walk a long journey without stilts, than a short one with them—say, for the sake of argument, three miles without stilts, than one mile with them ; then we come at once to the proof or reason why—one which is very plain, for at every step on stilts the pedestrian has to raise the whole weight of his body higher by muscular force than when on foot, and by muscles, too, not well adapted for the purpose as already stated (70), and upon which there must consequently be an extra amount of tear and wear daily. In addition to the extra force thus expended, he has also to counteract, by muscular force, a certain amount of reaction, and then to start from a comparative state of rest at every step. Now, such is just what the labourer experiences in walking in his rigid boots—that which makes him breathe hard, struggle and fight with both arms and legs in a painfully distressed manner, eat and drink double allowance to support the extra tear and wear upon the system, and so forth, and yet at the end of a ten-mile journey he is more fatigued and exhausted than his rival at the end of some thirty miles.

160. This peculiar stilting gait of the labourer, whose feet is thus fast in his rigid boots, will perhaps be better understood if we examine somewhat more closely the peculiar mechanism of his boot, and how closely it resembles the shoe of the engineer's rocking

lever, both having a convex sole. Boots of this kind are made upon a last having a convex sole, technically termed, in trade-phraseology, "*the spring of the last,*" so that the sole of the boot has a certain curvature like the tyre of a cart-wheel. The cart has two wheels, each forming a complete circle, so that they roll without any jolting action or break. The labourer has two boots and two legs—two felloes and two spokes, but, unfortunately, his two wheels are not complete; hence the upshot. But of this, more after in detail, when we come to soldiers marching, &c. (192—219).

161. The trained pedestrian, on the contrary, walks, to use a common expression, "with a light step," his outstretched foot in front touching the ground softly, and by means of its elastic movement, leaving it as gently behind. In his movements there is no jolting action from foot to foot—no hammering of hobnails against stones or other inequalities of the road—no concentration of forces antagonistically opposed to the common cause and course of progression—no reaction to counteract—no starting afresh at every step; for once in motion, he takes advantage of the momentum of his body, and, like the skilful skater on the ice, keeps going ahead with a uniform velocity and dignity of carriage, at a fraction of the expenditure of muscular force experienced by the labourer. In this how truly is "the poor man's case the poor man's lot"?

162. If the rigid lacing-boot is unsuited for the labourer after his foot has attained to maturity of growth, it is tenfold more so for youth, whose feet are growing. From what has been said in preceding sections (80—87), the reason of this need not be again told, for nothing can be more injurious than the rigid-soled boots in question, to the growing feet, and to the constitutional health generally of the young people that wear them. And what greatly increases the objectionable character of such boots, is the well-known fact, that at this period of life boys and lads, " if they have any life in them," or " are worth anything," are fond of trying each other's abilities at various athletic games and sports, such as foot-racing, jumping, and numerous feats of this kind, which test in the extreme the muscular strength of the foot and leg; consequently, many injuries are sustained under such circumstances, not unfrequently laying the foundation of constitutional debility experienced in after life. A high-spirited boy will strain every nerve and muscle to the utmost stretch before he is beaten by his rival; and when the right muscles are denied their natural freedom, and the wrong ones have to perform the extra work (70), the upshot is manifest. The playful exercise of this period of life is unquestionably a wise provision on the part of PROVIDENCE for the cultivation of constitutional health, and the proper development of every organ and member of the body—so that the foot-dress now

worn by the rising generation in our provinces is very far from what it should be. Indeed, it were difficult to conceive anything more fraught with unfavourable consequences to the physical well-being of our agricultural population.

163. The next example is what may not inaptly be termed "fashionable toes"—a boot or shoe with "a stylish toe," such as is now worn by a large proportion of the population in every rank of society. It were difficult, however, to imagine anything more unlike a comfortable covering for the toes of the human foot, than a stylish-toed boot. There appears to be something of an hereditary type about this fashionable toe; for in principle it was as great a favourite in Dr. Camper's time as at the present day. The statue of George IV., Trafalgar Square, and a thousand similar examples, prove how faithfully, in representing a fashionable-toed boot or shoe, artists have done their duty. It is made upon a last, shaped in front like a wedge—the thick part or instep of the last rising in a ridge from the centre or middle toe instead of the great toe, as in the foot, the last thus slanting off to both sides from the middle, terminating at each side and in front like a wedge—that for the inside or great toe being similar to that for the outside or little toe—as if the human foot had the great toe in the middle, and a little toe at each side, like the foot of a goose! Many fashions are, no doubt, very ridiculous when examined from

a common-sense point of view; perhaps, they have a right to a certain amount of latitudinarianism in this direction—be it so—and certainly foremost in the list may be ranked the "stylish toe" of boots and shoes, as now worn. That lasts and the boots and shoes made after this fashion can be manufactured more easily, and for less money, is possibly true—that they both "go sooner to the dogs," is equally susceptible of very easy proof—and that they are consequently a more profitable trade speculation, requires little to be said by way of demonstration; and when I have said this, perhaps I have told the simple reason why such a fashion is allowed to occupy so prominent a place in the shoeing of mankind.

164. "Trampling on one's toes" is a proverbial expression familiar to all, and in my experience I have oftener than once found the affair of "stylish toes" a very tender one. But, although existing prejudices and a certain amount of shortsighted selfishness may be deeply rooted in favour of the wedge-shaped toe of the last, and the corresponding form of the interior of the boot or shoe made upon it, yet facts must be left to speak for themselves; and the simple truth that must now be told is briefly this: However unlike the toes of the foot the toe of the last may be, yet into the place from whence the latter is taken by the shoemaker the former must be wedged by his customer!

165. This wedging of the toes into the acute angle of the interior of the toe of the boot or shoe formed by the wedge-shaped toe of the last is certainly without its parallel in the history of dress. There is no exaggeration in this; for the reader can hardly credit what observation daily calls upon us to acknowledge as fact, that an organism so delicately sensitive as the great toe of man, an inch and upwards, it may be, in thickness at the point, should be forced into the place, or acute angle, from whence the sharp edge of a wedge of wood has been taken! A circumstance so absurdly incredible, who can believe it? Yet such is the thickness of the toe, such the thickness of the last, and such the interior capacity of the toe of the boot or shoe!

166. The solution of the practical problem involved in this anomalous state of things will be found in the deformity of the toes of the foot, and in the corresponding change that takes place in the toe of the boot or shoe. In each case, a slow process of malformation takes place, commencing in childhood, in the former, and in the latter with every change of shape, size, &c., that takes place in the wearing and renewal of the boot or shoe, the point of the great toe and the point of the little toe being squeezed nearer and nearer to each other, until the former is brought into the line of the central metatarsus and its toe, as shown in Plate III.,

Fig. 4, while this growing deformity of the foot keeps continually twisting the shoe from bad to worse until it is thrown aside, when St. Crispin begins again to put on another wedge, as corns, bunions, and the other etceteras involved may suggest!

167. Were the deformity that takes place in the shape and position of the toes effected at once, as the blacksmith forges a piece of malleable iron, or as the last-maker shapes a piece of wood into a last, it could not be tolerated; but being a work of imperceptible degrees, it too often so happens that before the mind has arrived at a degree of maturity to form a correct judgment of the facts of the case, the work of metamorphosis, if not completed, has so far advanced as to render conclusions difficult to be arrived at, present appearances predicating so faintly what the original design was, and what the ultimatum may be as to the final shape of the toes. In short, it too frequently occurs that the rising generation are led astray by the force of fashion and the suavity of self-interested shoemakers, just at that period of life when they begin to act on their own account, the upshot being deformed toes. And to such an extent is this applicable, that it may not inaptly be said to be the rule rather than the exception; for at the meridian of life very few ever saw the normal form and position of their own toes, so as to be able to say positively, from observation, what they once were, what they may be, or what

they should be! After once deformity has taken place in infancy, riper years can, at the best, only form an opinion; and when we reflect how prone the opinions of fallen humanity are to run counter to the designs of an ALL-WISE CREATOR, it certainly becomes every one to weigh well and estimate cautiously the appeals of fashion, before they allow their minds to be biassed in favour of the slow process of deforming their feet.

168. With regard to the continual change that takes place in the wedge-shaped form of the toe of the boot or shoe in question during the lifetime of the wearer, little need be said on the matter, as the requirements of the healthy foot at different ages have already been noticed (83—88), and as the case of the diseased foot will subsequently be treated (Chap. XI.). It may, however, be proper to observe here, that the change in the toe of the shoe is not only one of those practical results demanded by the growing deformity of the toes, but also by the fact, that when once the work of deformity is begun, it must of necessity progress so long as a wedge-toed covering is worn, there being nothing to arrest its unhappy course, until the final dissolution of the body. This will appear manifest if we go back and trace the work from its commencement; for when the foot is growing, every new pair of boots must be a size larger than the old ones, as shown in the next section; but when the foot has attained to

maturity of growth, deformity does not then cease to make progress, but the contrary; for when once the meridian of life is passed, the evil work only progresses the faster, complaints becoming annually louder, more numerous and frequent, relative to the pinching of the toes demanding corresponding alterations in the form of the shoe by the shoemaker.

169. It is infancy and that period of youth during which boys and girls pay little or no attention to the proper growth and development of their toes that calls for special commiseration under this wedge-toed system of shoeing. If an elderly gentleman feels his corns, bunions, and inflamed toes more tightly wedged into the acute angle of the toe of his boots by the elongation of his foot than he concludes they should be, he grumbles very loudly in the ear of his shoemaker; pointing particularly in every direction, he imagines things are wrong, throws aside, it may be, the "misfits," and orders a new pair with more comfort; but the boots of the happy little boy, from being a size larger than the old ones, afford a temporary relief, and away he goes, jumping and prancing, delighted with the change; but by the time the uppers begin to get rigidly hard, his growing toes are up into the acute angle again, when the work of pinching and malformation by the elongation of his foot at every step begins afresh, each pair of new boots thus gradually moulding the growing foot into a deformed shape more successfully than the preceding pair, by a sort

of intermittent, yet, upon the whole, accelerated process!! A more vexatious, pain-producing system of shoeing youth, or one more ingeniously contrived and carried out for the malformation of the tender toes at this period of life, can hardly be imagined.

170. The toes in this deforming process are wedged into the toe of the boot horizontally and vertically, in the latter case the point of the great toe and little toe being forced nearer and nearer to each other, as already shown (166), and the joint of the great toe bent upwards, as stated by Dr. Camper, so as to force the point of the nail, as it were, to grow into the acute angle of the toe of the boot. But to avoid repetition, the details of the present shape of the toe of the boot and shoe, and the manner toes ride upon each other, will be noticed together in a subsequent chapter, when speaking of the restoration of the deformed foot to its normal shape (Chap. XI.)

171. The last example I shall notice in this chapter is " High heels," " *Military heels*," " Fashionable heels." The proposition, it will be seen, is a general one, applicable to boots and shoes having heels of a greater thickness than the rest of the sole. Although not worn of the same extreme height as in Dr. Camper's time, as shown in his drawings, fashionable high heels are still too common, and subject to all the objections he so ably advances against them, and something more.

172. In addition to what Dr Camper has said

against high heels, I shall briefly draw attention to two or three injurious results to which they, as at present constructed, give rise.

173. The high heel of the boot in raising the heel of the foot higher from the ground than the toes, places it and the whole body of the pedestrian in the same position as when standing on an inclined plane, or as in going down an inclination or hill, which is always a very fatiguing attitude for the muscles thus called into action, as explained under sections 54, 55, and 56. There is perhaps no attitude under which the tendons and muscles of the foot and ankle are more liable to be sprained or otherwise injured than in this; and the high heels, moreover, make every steep hill steeper than what it is, consequently more difficult to descend, and more liable to produce harm, without adding any counter avantage in going up-hill, as the heel of the nude foot, in such cases, does not touch the ground. In both cases, the high heel has, if possible, a worse feature than this, for it compels the knee to be lifted higher, as if stepping over a stone, which in going down-hill is always attended with danger to the foot.

174. In walking barefoot, as the weight of the body is gently brought forward, the heel rises from the ground, thus increasing the length of the radius without raising the body higher from the ground than in its erect position when standing, while in

the outstretched foot in front the other heel is raised upwards and the toes brought downward, so as to touch the ground softly, as formerly stated (161). Now it is manifest that if the heel of the boot raises the heel of the foot to the extreme height in walking, as shown in the case of walking barefoot, that the position is even more objectionable than walking on stilts, or in the rigid-soled lacing boots of the labourer (160), because it is subject to two objections instead of only one (159 and 173). And so on, the objection being proportionately less for any diminution in the height of the heel of the boot or shoe.

175. Again, in the high-heeled boot and shoe now made, the rigid "waist," with its triangular "shank-piece,"* which figures so prominently in their construction as a fashionable characteristic of elegance, has a considerable convexity inside, or upward curvature towards the underside of the arch of the foot ; and as it does not correspond therewith, it consequently forces up the key-stone of the arch, as it were, whenever the foot is subjected to any extreme pressure, thus weakening the whole of the structure and laying the foundation of a diseased or

* "Shank-piece," or "waist-piece," so called from its situation in the middle of the boot ; it is composed of one or more layers of very thick, hard, rigid leather, placed one above the other on the inner sole, forming an angle ; and when the outer sole is placed over this angle, the whole becomes one solid unbending mass.—See Plate III., fig. 3.

flat foot. It has been shown that the piers of the arch of the foot recede from each other like the ends of a carriage-spring (27), so that the length of the span and the curvature of the arch is continually changing. Now builders are familiar with the fact that if they are called upon to put centring into an arch to support it, it must not be of a less span than the arch itself, otherwise they will bring the fabric about their ears; yet this is the mechanical characteristic of the fashionable rigid waists now so generally worn along with high heels.

176. From each of these examples it will readily be seen that the boots and shoes of the present day are even, if possible, more objectionable than those of the time when Dr. Camper wrote upon the subject. Notwithstanding all the advances made in applied science generally, including, as already observed, the shoeing of the lower animals,—What, we may here pause to ask, has been done to improve the shoeing of mankind? What steps have been taken to divert the mind of the great mass of the people, in every rank of society, from the thraldom of an erroneous fashion relative to the general functions of the foot, and the normal form and position of the toes, so unfortunately interfered with by the peculiar style of the dress worn on the feet? Indeed, the advances made in the other branches of industry have rather exercised an injurious tendency in this, the shoeing of man; for by an increase of toil and labour in the

polluted atmosphere of our large towns, with the corresponding change that has taken place in our rural districts, the foot is subjected to a much greater degree of hardship than formerly, while its covering is less adapted to its physical well-being under such altered circumstances.

## CHAPTER IX.

### ON THE WELLINGTON AND BLUCHER.

177. Having in the preceding chapter briefly examined, *first*, the objectionable character of the rigid lacing boot now worn by the agricultural labourer, more especially in reference to the manner it interferes with the functions of the sole and posterior portion of the foot; *second*, how unsuited the fashionable wedged-shaped toes of boots and shoes are for the anterior portion of the foot; and, *third*, the manner high heels interfere with the attitude of the body and its muscular economy, I am now in a position to investigate somewhat more closely those details of a general character applicable to the boots and shoes now commonly worn by the great mass of the people; and as the Wellington and Blucher have been chosen by official authority as the articles best adapted for the public service, and as they may be taken as a fair representation of the principles demanding attention, I shall confine my remarks almost exclusively to them, taking "sealed patterns" of the "regulation boots," as worn in the army, for illustration.

178. According to the old proverb, "to find out

the seat of the disease, is to effect half its cure," and in this chapter it may be further premised that the object in view throughout is carefully to examine short-comings, with a view to improvement. I have already shown that neither Wellingtons nor Bluchers, as now generally made, are adapted for the requirements of the human foot in any of the ordinary vocations of industry, they being both subject to all the objections mentioned in the previous chapter; and if they are not adapted for ordinary wear, it is manifest they are tenfold less so for the public service, especially according to the present exigencies of the country and general progress of things, every day proving that the success of military tactics is becoming more and more dependant upon the physical well-being of the soldier's foot.

179. I shall then proceed at once to the solution of the shoemaker's question, why the sealed pattern army boot is not adapted for the soldier's foot. This I do with a view to ascertain the defects of the former, for the purpose of effecting their removal; and the requirements of the latter referred in a previous section (93) to this chapter. From a general point of view, there is no difference between the requirements of the soldier's foot and the foot of any other person similarly circumstanced, as every foot ought to enjoy the highest degree of physical well-being, including health, strength, and proper development, so that what has already been said in

PLATE III.

Fig. 1.

*a* ---- *b*

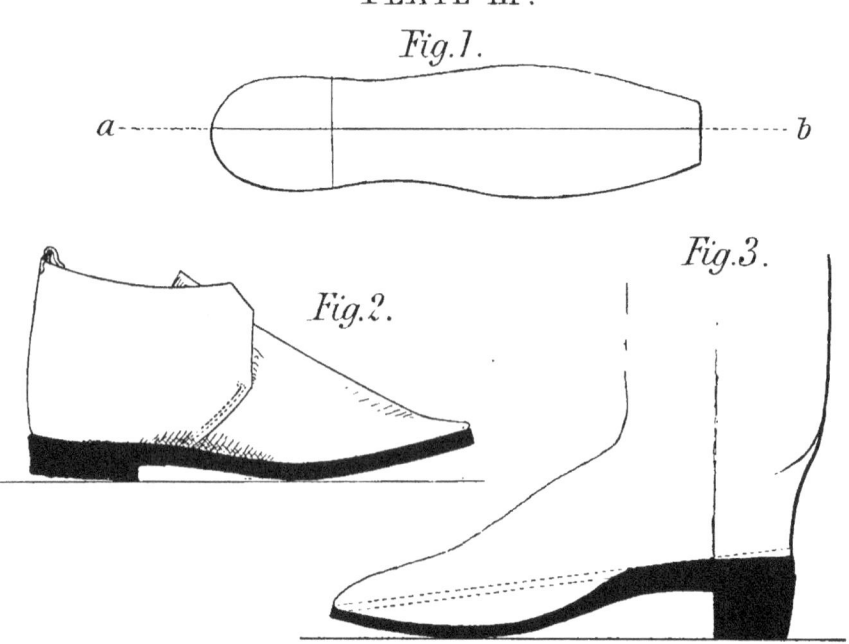

Fig. 2.

Fig. 3.

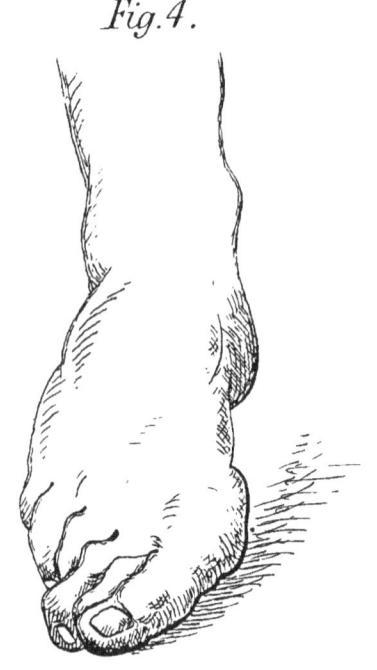

Fig. 4.

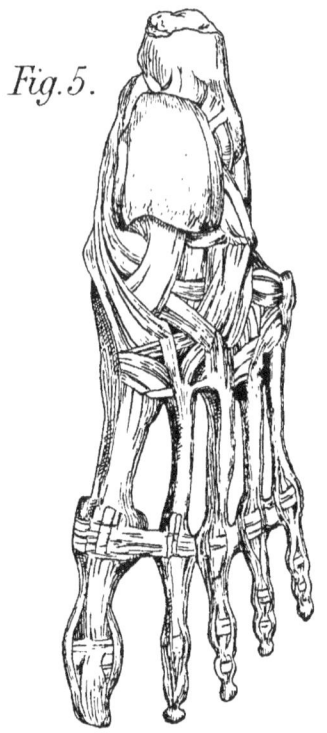

Fig. 5.

## WELLINGTONS AND BLUCHERS. 145

reference to the general health of the foot is applicable here. This will readily be granted, and for a similar reason the details about to be advanced here—details more especially demanded by the severe trials of military life, as the sequel will show—will be equally applicable to the extremes for which provision has to be made in all other cases (99). Notwithstanding all that may be said to the contrary, a proper foot-dress for the soldier is manifestly a great public question; and as such I shall endeavour to treat it, according to its practical merits

180. Plate III., Fig. 1, shows an outline of the sole of a sealed pattern army boot, a No. 8 Blucher; and Fig. 2, a side view of the same, both drawn to the same scale. There are seven sizes of patterns, 5, 6, 7, 8, 9, 10, 11, so that No. 8 is about a medium. Fig. 3 is a side view of a Wellington boot having a high heel and rigid waist; the form of the sole otherwise is similar to Fig. 1. Both boots are considered improvements on those worn during the war in the Duke of Wellington's time.

181. Both boots are made on wedge-toed lasts. The spring of the last in Fig. 2 is nearly an inch, and in Fig. 3 rather more. A straight line from the outer edge of the toe of the sole at $b$, Fig. 1, to the heel $a$, measures $11\frac{3}{8}$ inches, and gives a convexity or curvature of the sole of rather more than an inch. It is this latter curvature of the bottom

L

of the sole that gives to the rigid boot the peculiar characteristic of the rocking lever.

182. The sole, Fig. 1, is nearly straight, although intended to be worn on the left foot, a line, $a\ b$, passing through the middle of the heel to the middle of the toe, dividing the rest of the sole into two equal parts very nearly, so that it may be said to be exactly similar in principle in this respect to Fig. 8, Plate II., in Dr. Camper's drawings. The toe of the last, upon which the boot has been made, or the interior breadth of the sole at the toe, is 2 inches, terminating in an acute angle, owing to the toe of the last being of a wedge shape (See Sec. 186).

183. The thickness of the great toe varies in different individuals, as has already been shown (43), and the distance a soldier's toe can be forced into the acute angle of the wedge-toed boot in question will depend greatly upon the thickness of the bone, as the fleshy part can be compressed or flattened on the under or fleshy side, until the flesh separate and the skin be forced almost to touch the bone! But no great toe can be so flattened as to be forced into the toe of the army boot, Fig. 2, any more than it can be forced into the sheath of a sword, for it can only reach a certain distance, and no farther, without altering the configuration of the toe of the boot.

184. The forcing of the great toe into the toe of such a boot becomes, therefore, a practical question to the shoemaker,—one, too, of no ordinary im-

portance. In fitting a foot with a ready-made boot, as the one under notice, for example, the first thing that arrests his attention is, how far can the great toe be wedged into the acute angle of the toe of the boot from whence his last has been taken? What position will the point of the great toe occupy? Is the broad toe of the boot any improvement upon the narrow one of the old pattern, or those of Camper's time, represented in Plate II., Fig. 8? These and other kindred questions arise, demanding of him a practical solution.

185. Under measurement, it has been shown (105 to 109) that special provision requires to be made for the position, thickness, and curvature of the great toe, and toes generally, so as to preserve them in their natural form; and also, that the practical anomaly apparent on the surface of the first of these questions depends upon the extent to which the deforming process has been carried (166 to 170) in the distortion of the toes of the foot, and not unfrequently the anterior ends of the metatarsal bones (See Plate III., Fig. 4), and also in the stretching and disfiguration of the toe of the boot. In some cases, when this part of the foot is strong, the uppers may be stretched to allow the point of the toe to reach almost close to the extreme length of the boot; but in the vast majority of cases it is otherwise, the strong uppers resisting the strength of the toes, so that on examining the feet of soldiers,

and, indeed, the feet of all who wear such wedge-toed boots, there will invariably be found a considerable space in front, into which the point of the great toe cannot enter with the elongation of the foot.

186. With regard to the other two interrogatories, the point of the great toe will invariably be found nearly in the middle of the toe of the boot. This is effected by the joint agency of several causes; for, in the first place, the uppers stretch more easily and readily in the middle than towards the two sides, while the angles at the sides are nearly as acute as the one at the toe. Again, from this acuteness of the angle in front and on the two sides, it is manifest that the broad toe of the boot, under such circumstances, is no improvement upon the old pattern, or the narrow-toed shoes of Camper's time, but the reverse, the points of the toes being more liable to sustain injury from the elongation of the foot, wedging them at every step into the acute angle of the toe of the boot. If two boards or planed surfaces lie flat the one upon the other, there is no room between them to hold anything. So it is with rigid leather; for if a strong upper lies flat upon the sole, there is no space between them for the toes, let the breadth of the sole be what it may, unless by the wedging and stretching process. An extra breadth of sole at the toe of the boot, therefore, is no safe guide that suitable provision is made for the comfort of the great

toe. The truth of this will be seen when we consider that a sole one inch wide, with two inches of clear upper, will afford more room than "*a two-inch sole*" with only "a two-inch upper lasted on it." There ought just to be as great a difference between the toe of the soldier's boot and the sheath of his sword, as between his great toe and his sword.

187. Plate III., Fig. 4, gives an illustration of a foot deformed by the above wedging process. It is taken from the cast of a foot, and is therefore a genuine representation of injured toes. The point of the great toe, it will be seen, is brought to the middle of the toe of the boot, or to the line $A\ B$, Fig. 8, Plate II, and Plate III., Fig. 1, $a\ b$, being nearly in a line with the middle of the metatarsus. When in the boot, or even in the stocking only, the disfiguration is hardly perceptible; but what appears the most remarkable, is the fact, that in the eyes of the fashionable world it looks even more beautiful than when the toes are in their natural position! What would be the upshot were fashion to propose nude toes on high occasions is difficult to imagine; but one thing is plain, it is this: *the fashionable world would present the fewest fashionable feet.* The beauty of the human hand has long been among artists a subject of the highest interest; and as the foot occupies scarcely a less prominent position in physiological anatomy, why should it be so neglected as it is? What artist would think of putting

the above likeness (Fig. 4) on canvas, as a fair representation of the human foot?

188. But if the appearance of the nude foot looks unsightly, what are the actual consequences experienced by the soldier? Mr. Holden, in his work on "Human Osteology," says, "The last two phalanges of the little toe are generally anchylosed in adults, in consequence of being cramped in tight shoes, so different from that free spreading of the toes which Nature intended!" When a policeman, volunteer, or soldier is ordered to "stand at ease," he is simply called upon to exercise all the bones and muscles in his body, or nearly so; and of the numerous bones and muscles of the feet (see page 46), those more immediately employed in standing are by improper shoeing rendered inactive. How can he obey orders? In alluding to this topic, Paley says,—

"There is another property, more curious than it is generally thought to be, which is the faculty of *standing;* and it is more remarkable in two-legged animals than in quadrupeds, and, most of all, as being the tallest, and resting upon the smallest base in man. There is more, I think, in the matter than we are aware of. The statue of a man, placed loosely upon its pedestal, would not be secure of standing half an hour. You are obliged to fix its feet to the block by bolts and solder, or the first shake, the first gust of wind, is sure to throw it down. Yet this statue shall express all the mechanical properties of a living model. It is not therefore the mere figure, or merely placing the centre of gravity within the base, that is sufficient; . . . . the gift appears to me to consist in a faculty of perpetually shifting the centre of gravity, by a set of obscure, indeed, but of quick-balancing actions, so as to keep the line of direction within its prescribed limits. A man is seldom conscious of his voluntary powers in keeping himself upon his legs."

Such is the unanimous voice of Nature; but the "sealed pattern boot" of our Government completely reverses the design of an ALL-WISE CREATOR, leaving the poor soldier to reap the unfortunate consequences!

189. Before inquiring what those consequences experienced by the soldier are, let us examine first another very objectionable characteristic of this army boot, and all boots made on the same plan. We allude to the inner curvature of the sole, noticed in a previous section (175), and shown in Figs. 2 and 3, Plate III. It in some measure of necessity accompanies "high heels," "rigid waist," and "spring of the last." In a previous section (33), it has also been shown that the outside of the sole of the foot, from the heel to the little toe, touches the ground in the majority of cases when walking. When in repose, it may not be straight; but when the weight of the body is thrown upon the arch it is otherwise, nearly the whole outside then forming a straight bearing; under such circumstances what will the effect produced upon the lateral arch of the foot be, by its under side striking against the rigid curved waist of the sole at every step?

190. In following up the details of what was formerly said, principally in reference to the longitudinal

arch (173, 174, 175), the continual hammering of the bottom or outside pier of the lateral arch of the foot on the rigid curved sole will gradually beat down the objectionable curve itself, so as to bring it into the same plane or line with the heel—the posterior part of the sole inside being then straight from the heel to near the articulation of the little toe with its metatarsus. It is principally, therefore, in new boots that harm is done to the articulations of the bones of the posterior part of the foot. In some cases, however, the curve of the waist of the boot may be too strong to be beaten down straight by the lateral pier of a weak foot, so that in exceptions of this kind the foot will experience continual harm, the ultimate result being a rigid flat foot, if not something worse. If proper shoeing is had recourse to in time, as shown in another chapter (XI.), the injured foot may in many cases be restored to a comparative degree of soundness; but where the arch is entirely broken down, and a rigid flat foot experienced, the person is lame for life, being no longer able to walk as he formerly did, before the arch of his foot was broken down. The toes are now turned outwards, so that the foot stands at a right angle to the zigzag line, consequently the movement of each foot on to the other is sideways, with a lateral bending of the knee,—walking thus becoming a painful and laborious operation.

191. When the interior convexity of the waist

of the boot is reduced so as to relieve the outside pier of the lateral arch, the keystone of the longitudinal arch will then strike the top of the waist on the inside, until it is next reduced; and while this levelling of the curvature of the waist is being done, the sole of the boot will become a little elongated, and the toe turned upwards, thus increasing its distance from the ground. At the same time, the radius of the curvature of the sole or of the rocking lever will be reduced, while the uppers across the tread will be disfigured by creases and wrinkles, giving this part of the boot a very unsightly appearance, and rendering it extremely uncomfortable to the wearer when the leather gets hard, the bones and muscles not only sustaining injury from being kept in an unnatural position, but also inflamed by friction, &c., the muscles above and below losing their power of extension and contraction.

192. This increasing the height of the toe of the boot from the ground is tantamount to increasing "the spring of the last," and to reducing the radius of the rocking lever. These are facts that cannot be passed over superficially, as they involve practical questions, possessing, at the least, a certain value one way or another. Let us, therefore, examine them from a practical point of view.

193. When Robin Hood wished to send his arrow to a greater distance, he just bent his bow

so much the more, and in bending further the sole of our military boot, and thus *increasing* "*the spring of the last*," is it thereby understood in military tactics that the soldier in marching will spring further? To me there has always been something anomalously perplexing in the very expression "spring of the last," considering that a last is perfectly non-elastic, so to speak; for does not the sole of the last resemble more the foot of a child's cradle, or "rocking-horse," than any sort of a spring? Engineers have certainly been more fortunate in the technical phraseology of a "rocking lever;" for this unquestionably involves the action of the foot when walking in the rigid-soled boot in question; and it is equally manifest that the shorter the radius of the foot of the child's cradle or rocking-horse, the more easily is it rocked; and just so is it with the rigid-soled military boots of the present day. The soldier in marching rocks more easily in his boots the more they are curved in the sole: unfortunately, however, as we increase the spring of the last, we at the same time increase his stilting gait when the drum beats an equal length of step—hence the inevitable upshot.

194. In discussing this peculiar and undignified stilt-stilting and *trampling* gait of our soldiers in marching, and also of all others who wear rigid-soled boots, it will be necessary to notice more closely the mechanical details of walking than was

done in previous sections (23, 156 to 161), to which reference is made. It was there shown that the line of progression was zigzag (23); that the lacing boot of the agricultural labourer compelled him to walk with a stilting gait, quoting Sir Charles Bell in support of what was there said (159) as to the contrast between rigid-soled shoeing and the reverse, while under (161) the advantages gained by the trained pedestrian walking in easy shoes were shown. We shall now endeavour to show the reason why the losses were sustained in the one case and the advantages gained in the other.

195. Were it possible to examine each foot separately, under an old hypothesis, that progression is rectilinear, then according to this beautiful theory of walking, two carriage-wheels on their axles furnish a good illustration of the principle involved; and if we further suppose the length of the leg or radius 3 feet, and the step or pace 3 feet, these data would give us a wheel 6 feet in diameter; with three soles or shoes upon each wheel, so placed that the footprint of each sole on the one wheel would be 3 feet from the respective footprints on the other wheel. Again, if it is further granted, as is the case according to this old theory, that the soles in each wheel are in the same vertical plane, *i. e.*, that the line A B, Fig. 8, Plate II., and *a b*, Fig. 1, Plate III., is in each case in the line of progression, or in the middle

of the tire of the wheel, then we get rid of "out-toes" and "in-toes," "going over the sole," sometimes on the outside, at other times on the inside; the rotary motion of the line $a\,b$ in each sole being rectilinear. But it need hardly be added that this unfortunately does not illustrate the true theory of walking, that with which the shoemaker has to deal. But nevertheless two wheels on a common axle, with three spokes each—each spoke with its felloe or sole rotating along the road, would illustrate very forcibly the rocking gait of the soldier in marching, although perhaps somewhat extravagantly, owing to the absence of flexion at the knee, with some other differences of detail needless to notice.

196. Advantage has been taken of the above old theory in the manufacture of several very popular toys amongst children, representing soldiers and others moving along on wheels; and, however absurd may be the extreme distance to which the proposition is thus carried, it only serves the more forcibly to prove the impropriety of leaving the natural path of truth, so to speak, and entering upon that of error in the shoeing of man. In other words, it proves very forcibly the absurdity of changing the natural character of the leverage of the human foot and leg, by converting them into that of a rocking lever, through the instrumentality of rigid-soled boots and shoes.

197. The foot and leg of man form an elastic self-elongating system of leverage, so to speak, differing in many respects from a rocking lever. The nude foot in walking, for example, does not rock on the ground from heel to toe like the foot of a child's cradle or the fulcrum end of a rocking lever, much less is the movement from one foot to the other of a jolting character. The reverse of this is true, as has already been shown (161) ; and I shall now endeavour, as briefly as possible, to show the principal differences between the two systems, pointing out the advantage of the one and disadvantages of the other.

198. In the example of a pedestrian already quoted (161) whose feet and legs are, by proper training, in the highest degree of health, strength, and elasticity for successful walking, the body advances nearly at a uniform motion, rising and falling very little, horizontally, from the line of progression, while, vertically, its zigzag motion from foot to foot is much less than in the case of the soldier marching in rigid Bluchers, the line of progression being of a somewhat different character.

199. This uniform even motion is produced by the elasticity of the foot and elongation of the radius or leg by the outstretching of the instep in front and behind, thus presenting a threefold attitude of body, a mean and two extremes, deserving of special attention.

200. In both the extremes, or cases of elongation before and behind, the increase in the length of the radius is considerable, while, when the body is passing over the one foot to the other no elongation takes place, but the reverse, owing to the flexion at the knee.

201. The position of man in walking may thus be represented by a right-angled triangle, A B C; the length of the step A B being the base; the length of the leg B C, at the moment the line of gravitation coincides with it, being the perpendicular; and the outstretched leg behind A C being the hypotenuse: or, expressed in other terms, B C may be the radius, A B the tangent, and A C the secant of the angle A C B, or angle made by the two legs A C and C B in walking— what may not unaptly be termed *the natural step*.

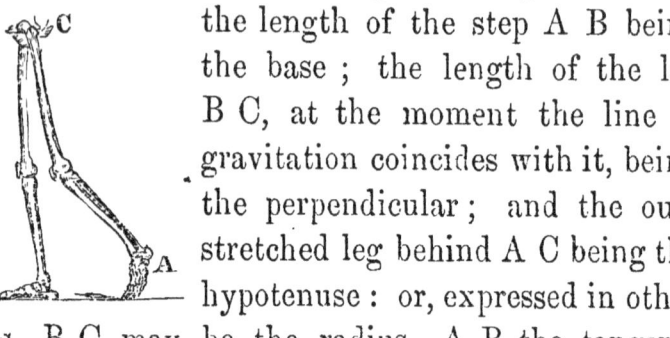

202. As to muscular elasticity, the moment the line of gravitation passes the foot as the body in its onward course advances, then its whole weight is supported by this elasticity or muscular force, now being exerted in the work of elongating the lever from the length of the radius to that of the secant, while the secant in front is as gradually changed into the radius when the weight of the body is thrown upon it.

203. It will thus be seen that it is the gradual

elongation of the leg or radius by the contraction of the muscles of the calf of the leg and those of the sole of the foot, thereby bringing the instep into nearly a line with the leg at the moment the toe behind is leaving the ground, that keeps the body advancing at a uniform motion and at a uniform distance from the ground.

204. The free exercise of this elasticity of the foot is of still greater importance when the pedestrian is called upon to take a longer step than his natural one above (201), as in a quick march—running, jumping, and the like, as the extra length of step has to be effected by this muscular force. The swiftness of some Indians, the ease with which they run, and the peculiar configuration and muscular movements of their feet, may be quoted as practical illustrations of this.

205. On the other hand, the foot of the soldier, when tightly laced into a rigid Blucher, is deprived of this elasticity and consequent power of elongating the leg from the radius to the secant in marching; strictly speaking, in his case there is neither tangent nor secant, but only two radii of equal length—or "spokes of the wheel," as they have been termed—the two elastic self-elongating levers formerly mentioned (197, 201) being metamorphosed into two rocking ones (196) in degree according to the rigidity of the boot, the muscular strength to bend the sole, and the tightness of the lacing of the boot.

206. Our next proposition, therefore, is the *modus operandi* of rocking from one foot to another in walking. From what has been said, it will now be seen that when the line of gravitation passes the foot, the body is gradually lowered, until the next foot touches the ground, when it again gradually rises, so that at every step it describes a curve. This is a characteristic so different from the even, uniform motion in the opposite case (201), that it demands special attention, for the momentum of the body has now a centrifugal action around the fulcrum on which it thus turns, so that the foot must come bumping against the ground at every step. It is this bump-bumping that gives to the tread of soldiers in marching its peculiarly rocking and undignified trampling character, so destructive to pontoons, bridges, and everything under their feet; so that it is more than probable that a thousand Indians would cross ice that would not carry a hundred British soldiers! But be that as it may, it is manifest that this trampling is very injurious to both boots and muscles; the former suffering from concussion against the ground, by the centrifugal force of the body; and the latter, from the reaction which is thus of necessity experienced. It is not only trying for both the boot and the foot, when they touch the ground in front, but also in starting afresh at every step from a state of com-

parative rest—for the body has to be raised by a sudden effort of the muscles to the level from whence it descended, so that the boot again suffers against the ground, and the muscles, by this unnatural extra exertion. Hence the heavy plodding gait of all who wear boots of this kind.

207. But this is not all with the soldier; unfortunately for him, he has to carry his knapsack and accoutrements, and march in all climates, with his feet thus imprisoned in his "regulation boots," depriving them of their natural functions; and when it is borne in mind that the additional weight of his knapsack and other accoutrements, amounting to some 60lbs., is carried at the extreme of a long leverage from the foot, thus greatly increasing the momentum with which the latter must strike the ground, and the muscular force required to raise the whole to the natural level, his condition may be more easily imagined than described.

208. The exact rise and fall of the body will depend upon the length of the leg and step, and the centrifugal force of the knapsack to the height of the soldier; but these are details into which it is not my province to enter.

209. A parallel example, however, may just be mentioned, viz., the steam-engine. In this case, the engineer can tell the force of steam required to raise any given weight, the extra height to which the soldier has to raise himself, and also

the expense per mile in travelling; and a very small amount of reflection must convince every impartial reader, that the extra tear and wear to which the muscles of the soldier are subject in marching to the battle-field to fight for his country, under the burning sun of China or India, and under all the exciting influences of an active campaign, must be something very considerable.

210. We now come to examine the zigzag movement of the soldier, and why it is greater than in the case of the trained pedestrian, with his light elastic shoe—the sepoy (see foot-note, 93), with his sandal, or the Indian barefoot; although otherwise he may be much the superior of the three as to muscular strength generally.

211. The articulations of the foot admit of a lateral as well as a hinge movement in walking, but the rigid regulation boots of the army deprive the foot of both, if not wholly, in many cases, to a very great extent.

212. Deprived of these movements, the foot also loses that beautiful and absolutely necessary provision in the elastic expansibility of the lateral arch, already noticed in a previous section (44), that gives stability of posture (188), as well as safety to the bones of the foot and leg in walking.

213. Instead of the soldier's foot turning upon its natural articulations under such conditions, the sole of the boot now turns upon the ground with

a grinding action, like a pestle in a mortar; and it is this grinding action that proves so destructive to the thick, hard, rigid sole as already noticed (141).

214. Under these circumstances the centre of gravity has to be brought more perpendicularly upon the foot at every step, in order to maintain an equilibrium of posture, when the heel comes bump against the ground, so as to be able to turn successfully the angles of the zigzag line or path, and also to perform the short rocking motion that takes place as the weight rocks from the heel to the toe, or until it gets another centrifugal hitch diagonally across to the other foot, grinding the sand and pebbles under the tread of the sole.

215. It is otherwise under the free muscular action of the nude foot, the body being then deflected, as it were, gently, from one foot diagonally to the other by the elasticity of the articulations, the centre of gravity of the body thus moving in a curved or waved line, rather than in a zigzag one. The momentum of the body has not now to turn sharp angles from one direction to another when it enters upon the field of the foot, so to speak, but in a curved line corresponding to something like the semi-domelike curvature of the lateral arch of the foot (49), apparently designed for this express purpose. There is something in these beautiful movements deserving of a more detailed notice than falls to the pen of a shoemaker to give.

216. Much of all this will depend upon how the boot fits, and the muscular strength of the foot to bend the sole. Although a regiment of soldiers may be trained to march with equal step, and although all the men may have been carefully selected, so that every foot in a draft of raw recruits is sound, there must, nevertheless, be in every corps a considerable diversity in the movements of different feet, owing to peculiar configuration of the foot, how the boot fits, with the tightness it is laced, and so forth. We have shown, for example, that feet are very different as to shape, irrespective of size; but there is no difference in the shape of the regulation boots of the army, generally speaking, the only difference being in the size; so that in a whole regiment a proper fit will rather be the exception than the rule. There is something so anomalously absurd in the fitting of army boots, when examined from a practical point of view, as to demand a passing notice; for as there are only seven sizes of pattern boots, the regulation obviously presupposes that all the feet in the army had been cast, as it were, in seven moulds!

217. These remarks relative to a proper fit are equally applicable to all who wear ready-made boots and shoes, and who, probably, upon the whole, do not fit themselves much better than infantry soldiers do generally.

218. This anomaly no doubt arises from the fact,

that when Bluchers are made more in conformity to the current fashion of the day than to the form of people's feet, the selection of a new boot is perhaps more influenced by the former than the latter. But be this as it may, it is manifest that so long as wedge-toed boots of the present fashion are the rule, a proper fit must of necessity be the exception. This part of the subject, however, falls to be discussed in another chapter (XII.), under trade systems, &c.

219. What has thus been said of the Blucher is equally applicable to the Wellington, with this difference, that the army pattern has a " shank-piece "* expressly put in by stipulation, to make it, if possible, more rigid and unbending at the waist than the Blucher! so that the objections to the whole may be thus summed up :—1. The rigidity of the waist atrophies the muscles of the foot and leg (156 and 157). 2. The inner convexity of the waist weakens both the longitudinal and lateral arches of the foot (174 and 175). 3. The spring of the last, or curva-

---

* " The insoles to be composed of crop shoulder insoles, English tannage. The shank-pieces to be equal in every respect to those attached to the pattern boots."—*Specifications for the Supply of Boots for the Royal Artillery. War Office, Pall Mall,* 1857.

To readers not acquainted with trade technicalities, I may mention, " shoulder insoles " are more rigid and unbending than " belly " or " flank ;" and the " shank-pieces " specified above are in thickness $\frac{3}{4}$ of an inch, so that when placed between the insole and outsole the total thickness of the waist will be from $1\frac{1}{4}$ to $1\frac{1}{2}$ inch. (See note on section 175.)

ture of the sole, gives rise to a rocking motion, and consequently to a centrifugal force or jolting gait, greatly retarding progression and increasing the consumption of muscular force (158, 206). 4. The bending or turning of the toe of the boot upwards also injures the muscles of the sole by continuous extension, and those above by continuous contraction (191). 5. The fleshy part of the great toe is a natural protection to the bone ; so that by the wedging and flattening process the bones of the toe are deprived of this natural protection, and the same applies to the other toes, the result being anchylosis (183 and 188). 6. The cramping of the toes and metatarsus destroys the elasticity of the foot, prevents the elongation of the lever or leg, and throws an extra amount of work upon other parts of the system, thus deranging the natural equilibrium of the whole (211 and 212). 7. High heels destroy the natural level of the foot and the proper attitude of the body. " By raising one pier, *i. e.* the heel-bone," says Mr. Holden, " we are always walking upon an inclined plane ; we alter the natural bearings of all the other bones ; we throw more pressure than Nature intended on the toes ; hence distorted feet, crooked toes, bunions, corns, *et id genus omne!*" (173 and 214). 8. And lastly, by destroying the natural play of the internal mechanism of the foot, we destroy at the same time the general health of the body ! (59.) Is it therefore to be wondered at, that footsore soldiers should fill our hospitals, and swell the mortality of every campaign in the manner they do? that in the French war Napoleon I. and his Generals should have always expressed so much concern about, and placed so high a value upon the health of the soldier's foot?—that all our own Generals and Military writers should take the same view of the subject;* and that our soldiers themselves should throw off their unbendable foot-gear, and charge the enemy barefoot,† or march with their boots at the muzzles of their guns instead of on their own extremities?‡ These are facts that speak for themselves, and the reasons we have adduced are more than sufficient to account for them!

* "The ammunition boots are villanous affairs: the leather is bad, the workmanship is bad, and the boot itself is wholly unfitted from its shape for these snows and this season of the year. When the plain was covered with adhesive viscid mud it separated the seams, and made openings between the layers of the soles; as the snow melts the leather soaks up the water, and in the morning the boot is frozen, and so hard that the soldier cannot get his swollen and tender foot into it. The number of men going to hospital is greatly increased by affections of the feet."—Letter dated Above Sebastopol, January 5.—*Daily News*, Jan. 26, 1855.

† Gen. Sir Robert Dick used to tell that when a Highland Regiment was at the battle of Maida, on being ordered to charge the enemy, all the soldiers took off their regulation-shoes and charged bare-footed.

‡ It is well known to those who have been in the West Indies that the West India regiments, composed of men of colour, invariably, when ordered to "march out," take off their regulation-boots and tie them together, and suspend them from the muzzle of their muskets.

## CHAPTER X.

ELASTICATED LEATHER—ITS OBJECT AND VALUE IN THE MANUFACTURE OF BOOTS AND SHOES.

220. It is now nearly thirty years since the idea first occurred to me of introducing into boots and shoes some elastic material to accommodate the foot in its ever-varying form in walking. Previous to this, the injured feet of many of my customers, coupled with their solicitous demands, for which the ordinary leather used in the manufacture of boots and shoes made no satisfactory provision, had very forcibly arrested my attention, forcing upon me the conclusion at which I ultimately arrived relative to caoutchouc, having, about the year 1830, purchased a quantity of the "native caoutchouc goloshes," then introduced for the first time from South America. In short, I then saw clearly a principle which I at once set about reducing to practice.

221. After several years' experimenting, with not a few failures, I succeeded in making a pair of boots for myself, having caoutchouc waists and gussets. The experiment gave so much promise of comfort in the wear, and healthy action to the feet, that I was induced to lay the subject before Sir John Robison,

President of the Royal Scottish Society of Arts, for a scientific opinion.

222. Sir John not only approved of the principle, but was so well pleased with the progress made in its reduction to practice, that he ordered an experimental pair of boots for himself, and some for several members of his family. But here I had the mortification to meet with another failure,—the action of the oil of the curried leather having destroyed the caoutchouc, where the two were joined in the gusset of the uppers, so that they separated the one from the other, after only a few days' wear; Sir John, however, found the beneficial effects of an elastic waist; and as the caoutchouc stood firm in the sole, he expressed a hope that it might be retained, the improvement thus far being highly satisfactory.

223. It was then I made the discovery of elasticated leather. Instead of being cast down and discouraged by the above failure, I felt the reverse; for from Sir John's experience harmonizing with my own, I became more sensibly alive than ever to the necessity of some elasticated material being introduced into the soles of boots and shoes; and although it cost me again several years' industrious experimenting, I still cherished, with increasing fondness, my discovery, and ultimately succeeded in reducing to practice the proposition of elasticating leather. In other words, in order to obtain a material having the property of expansibility and contractility, I in-

corporated the fibrous portion of skins with caoutchouc, in such a manner as to preserve for the fabric the tenacity and durability of the former, and the elasticity of the latter.

224. Elasticated leather is thus manufactured of the skins of animals and caoutchouc, the raw materials being first prepared for uniting to form the proper quality of fabric. Manufacturers have long been familiar with the art of weaving mixed fabrics of wool, flax, cotton, silk, &c. &c., the woof and warp being diversified in many different ways, according to pattern. They have also long been acquainted with the manufacture of "oil-cloth," "wax-cloth," and the endless variety of articles of this kind now in the market. In like manner my proposition was something similar to the latter class of articles in character, *my fabric being caoutchouc leather.* I required, for example, a fibrous texture of the strongest and most durable kind, on the one hand: this I found in the skins of animals; and also, on the other hand, an elastic material, which I found in india-rubber. I then had to unite the two substances together, so as to produce fabrics of various qualities, possessing all the characteristics of the originals as to durability and elasticity.

225. Elasticated leather can thus be manufactured of endless variety, according to the quality and preparation of the skin, and the quantity and quality of prepared caoutchouc, with which it is

## ELASTICATED LEATHER. 171

incorporated. It can be made of any thickness, from that of the strongest sole leather to that of the finest uppers; and the latter can be made sufficiently porous to permit the escape of perspiration, more so, I am convinced, than uppers generally, especially when filled with grease, or any of the numerous "repellents" now used for keeping out water.

226. As to the preparation of the raw materials, the fibrous texture of skins requires not only to be made sufficiently pure and porous, but so crimpled and contracted as to permit of the proper elongation required when incorporated with the caoutchouc. In this respect, the contraction of the fibres resembles in some measure, the contraction of live muscle. Indeed, the grand problem I had to solve was to make a material capable of expanding and contracting, to accommodate the contraction and expansion of the muscles of the foot; and to this extent the fibrous texture of skins requires to be contracted as a preparatory process in the manufacture of elasticated leather. As to the preparation of caoutchouc, nothing requires special notice.

227. My success in elasticated leather induced me, upwards of twenty-three years ago, to make an elastic sandal-tie or ribbon, the woof of which was common thread, and the warp threads of india-rubber. At that time sandal shoes, or slippers, were tied by means of ribbons around the ankle and crossing on the instep; they were much worn by ladies; and my

elastic sandal-ribbon was experienced to be a great improvement upon the common one. Since then its use has been much extended for gaiters, hatbands, glove-bands, &c. &c. Woven fabrics of a similar character are also now largely and successfully used as gussets in the uppers of boots and shoes; while improved patterns in silk, &c. are being used for the entire uppers.

228. Of the strength and durability of elasticated leather a doubt cannot now be fairly raised, as more than twenty years' experience has pronounced an unqualified award in its favour; it being now worn by all classes and ages of the community, proving itself without an exception more durable than the best sole leather.

229. It also stands any change of temperature in the weather, being equally eligible for summer and winter wear. But perhaps the best test of its quality in this respect is the fact, that it has been worn successfully amongst the perpetual snows of the Polar regions and the burning plains of India, and that it has been found in both cases more durable and better adapted to the comfort of the foot than the best leather.

230. I must here, however, remind my readers that it is the principle of elasticating leather and other materials used in the manufacture of boots and shoes that I have to discuss in this chapter, rather than the extent to which I have successfully reduced that

principle to practice. Between the two propositions there may be, and doubtless is, a wide difference, and therefore, without asking for myself more credit than what is due, *the* principle itself is, beyond all doubt, invaluable, involving one of the most important improvements connected with the foot-dress of man. Experimental inquiry is now abroad in this long-neglected but promising field, and too much encouragement cannot be given to the cause. Were I, and others practically engaged in the investigation of this movement, to study selfishly our own private interests only, our maxim would assuredly be to keep our secrets to ourselves; but the times in which we live are, it is hoped, ahead of such a spirit, the only open course now left for all being to put an honest shoulder to the wheel of progress.

231. With regard to the extent to which elasticated leather may be used in the manufacture of boots and shoes, a detailed account of my own practice alone would do more than fill this work from beginning to end. In this department I leave the matter almost entirely in the hands of my customers; but, generally speaking, an elastic waist only is ordered. Of late years, however, a demand for more has been gaining ground—some now wearing an entire innersole from heel to toe of elastic material—others the entire uppers of woven elastic fabrics, besides an elasticated leather waist, and so on—some one way, some another; moreover, in a country like this,

where so many feet are injured, as already noticed, by fashionable-toed boots and shoes, much depends upon the sanitary condition of feet, which brings me to my next chapter.

## CHAPTER XI.

### ON INJURED FEET, AND THEIR SANITARY IMPROVEMENT.

232. Ever since I laid my proposition of elasticated leather before the public, it has received the warmest patronage of the medical profession. A very large per-centage of the ills of fallen humanity are unquestionably traceable to the sad mismanagement of the lower extremities; and this is, no doubt, the reason why the family doctor, as well as professors of medical science in our universities, have supported the emancipation of the foot of man from the slavery of rigid leather.

233. Where the normal symmetry of the foot has been injured by the wedge-toed, rigid-soled, high-heeled boots and shoes now so commonly worn, it may, in a great many cases, if not the majority, be restored to its original beauty and health, by removing the cause of injury, so as to enable the foot to perform its natural functions. From being a living animal organism, the foot is subject, on the one hand, to a daily waste, and on the other hand, to a reparation or building up process; and in this daily rebuilding of the foot, Nature, if left unre-

strained, will restore it to its original shape; for she is not instigated by the caprice of fashion to grow crooked toes, or any of the many deformities produced by improper shoeing.

234. It is no easy matter, however, to remove wholly the cause that has given rise to crooked toes. When once the feet have been deformed by bad shoeing, it takes some considerable time to restore them to their original shape, however well the work of shoeing may be performed, because crooked toes are not pulled down and built up again every day. We may co-operate with Nature, and even assist her greatly, but we cannot grow crooked toes straight, as we grow cucumbers; the two operations being totally different. We can, no doubt, throw aside the wedge-toed, high-heeled, unyielding boots, and put on elastic ones; but we cannot throw aside so easily the distorted muscles, tendons, ligaments, and bones of the foot. This is Nature's own particular work, and although certain of performance at so much per day, regularly, when health is attended to, it is of necessity a slow one, because a series of renewals are often necessary before the original likeness is wholly attained.

235. In the case of healthy, robust constitutions, however, the length of time required to restore the feet to their original symmetry and beauty is often less than could well be calculated upon, and generally so flattering, from the compressed and flattened

fleshy parts soon assuming the round, plump shape of Nature, that the majority "enjoy the thing amazingly" (to use a rather common phrase). But of course it is otherwise with indifferent constitutions, or those engaged in unhealthy occupations.

236. A few practical examples will best illustrate what has further to be said on this subject. *First*, on injuries of the instep or arch of the foot; *second*, injuries of the toes, and their articulations; and *third*, injury to the anterior ends of the metatarsal bones. These, and a short account of how they are restored to a healthy state, will constitute the remainder of this chapter.

237. The arch of the foot very frequently sustains injury in childhood, before the bones and the cartilaginous members that unite them, as seen in the woodcut page 46, have become sufficiently firm and strong to support the weight of the body. And even after they have acquired the necessary strength, as when they have arrived at maturity of growth in manhood, they are frequently injured by improper shoeing. Many fine, healthy, strong, full-grown, well-arched feet are so injured by high heels, rigid soles, and convex waists (174, 175, 190), that they become flat-soled. Examples of this kind are numerous amongst our police and soldiers, men whose feet have been at one time examined and pronounced free from this

deformity, a flat sole being a disqualification of fitness for the public service.*

238. The latter two examples merit special notice. They do so for more reasons than one; for in the first place, the two parties are public servants, chosen and selected men, whose special duty imperatively requires that they should be qualified to endure hardship and fatigue. And in the second place, the injury is sustained under circumstances requiring to be more clearly understood than we fear it is in the responsible quarters of the Government, or perhaps we may say such lameness is produced by causes not generally dreamt of as being capable of effecting such results. The former of these propositions will be described in the next chapter, the latter only in this.†

* The following is contained in the 14th section of the Army Medical Instructions, as causes for the rejection of recruits :— " Impaired or inadequate efficiency of one or both of the inferior extremities on account of varicose veins, old fractures, malformation, flat feet, &c.; palsy or lameness, contraction, mutilation, extenuation, enlargement, unequal length, bunions, overlying or supernumerary toes, ganglions, &c., &c."—War Office, 30th July, 1830.

† So important is this deformity considered as unfitting men for the public service, that Gorcke, the Director-General of the Army Medical Department in Prussia, in a letter to the medical officers, dated July, 1818, states that " the remote and proximate causes of this deformity are still but very imperfectly known, and it is therefore much to be wished that army medical officers would avail themselves of every opportunity which offers to investigate the subject. To do this effectually, deformed feet

239. The continuous beat of policemen and soldiers, although the step may be slow, is very liable to produce lameness of the kind in question, viz., flat-foot. No better authority can be quoted in support of this, than G. Borlase Child, Esq., Surgeon-in-Chief to the City of London Police, and to the Royal London Militia, &c., who authorises me to say that his professional experience confirms its truth, he having always cases on hand. The arch of the foot is in such instances completely broken down by the continuous action of the convexity of the waist (174, 175, and 190). This is more rapidly effected when the general health has been impaired by cramped toes, &c. (59), as this prevents the rebuilding of healthy structure. The feet of the policeman and soldier thus become gradually weaker and weaker, and less able to bear fatigue. In both these cases, a very large per-centage of lameness is produced by the regulation boots of the public service, a few years' wear rendering men unfit for duty.

240. In examples of this kind, the advantages derived from wearing elastic boots and shoes are simply those accruing from the free exercise of the injured parts of the arch, exercise being essentially necessary to enable Nature to throw off waste refuse,

should not only be carefully inspected, but the parts of the feet ought to be examined after death. By this means we may be able to attain greater certainty in regard to the cause of the deformity, and perhaps to discover a rational plan of treatment."

and to produce a healthy growth and reparation,— the consequent gradual restoration of the muscles, tendons, and ligaments to a healthy state of action, with the gradual replacement of the bones of the arch, each bone having its bearings restored and properly lubricated. Protected externally, and left to the free play of its internal mechanism, the work of improvement once fairly begun, advances gradually to completion.

241. Crooked unsightly toes are just as common as fashionable wedge-toed boots and shoes; so that it may be said, without exaggeration, that perfect symmetry is of rare occurrence. More numerous examples of deformity, however, are to be found amongst broad thin feet, as already noticed (43), especially where the front angle is obtuse, the point of the little toe reaching nearly as far forward as the first joint of the great toe, the point of the latter being in this class of feet very often thick (46). The reason of this liability to lameness in toes of this class is manifest; the toes being levers, the longer they are the more easily bent, consequently the two extremes (the points of the great toe and little toe) have further to be brought towards each other in order to form the fashionable angle in front than in narrow feet, as will be seen in comparing Fig. 4 with Fig. 5, Plate III.; so that the articulations at the root of the great toe and little toe are opened on the outside and too closely compressed

on the inside, and as this wedge-shaped opening fills up it forms a false bearing, which has to be removed gradually before the toes can be restored to their natural position. The two principal joints thus become injured, while the intervening toes are squeezed into all sorts of shapes and positions. The illustration (Fig. 4) is an example of this kind, and Fig. 5, that of a healthy uninjured foot, showing the muscles or tackle (57).

242. But when the toes are thus distorted, it is seldom that the work of malformation ends here, the anterior extremities of the metatarsal bones also suffering harm, sometimes by being forced further asunder, thus spreading the articulations at the bend of the foot, and making it broader than it should be. This outspreading of the roots of the toes and ends of the metatarsal bones to which they are hinged, is effected partly by the pressure on the points of the toes from the elongation of the foot, and partly by the outward pressure of the other toes when squeezed together in front. There is, under such circumstances, a very unnatural jerking of the bones of the toes and those of the metatarsus at every step in walking, cruelly painful when the articulations become inflamed, as they very frequently do. In the other example the foot becomes narrower at the tread than it should be, owing to the middle metatarsal bones being forced down at the anterior extremities, and the two outside ones up; the points of both the great

toe and little toe very often riding across the others, thus forming a hollow above like the palm of the hand,—with the reverse a lateral curvature of the sole. This is also a most injurious deformity, as it destroys the stability of the base, or "footing," by undermining, as it were, the outside pier of the lateral arch in front, thereby producing a tendency to go over the sole to the outside.

243. It was formerly shown (27—29) that the foot in walking was subject to elongation in a twofold manner; this elongation being, in the one case, on the principle of a spring, and in the other, on that of a hinge. It has also been shown (142, 143) that an elastic waist in the boot or shoe made provision for these changes in the length of the foot; and we have now to consider how far this elasticity in the sole of the boot or shoe makes provision for injured toes and other deformities of this part of the foot, adding to those just mentioned (139, 140), corns, bunions, *et id genus omne.*

244. In the generality of cases, it is the elongation of the foot at every step, jerk-jerking the toes into the acute angle of the wedge-toed boot, that produces the most harm; and when relieved of this by the elongation of the sole at the waist, and when the muscles, tendons, ligaments, and bones begin to enjoy their natural free play within the boot, the foot in the first example (139) begins

to grow longer and narrower at the tread, often so rapidly in the case of those whose general health is good, and whose feet are, comparatively speaking, healthy, as very much to surprise them; so much so, that if the boot is made upon the old last, it will be too short and too wide at the tread: while in the second case (140), the foot becomes longer and broader. To those who have paid any attention to the anatomy of the feet, a moment's reflection must be sufficient to satisfy them of the reason of such changes; viz., that they are accounted for by the gradual restoration of the toes and bones of the metatarsus to their normal form and position. In this work of reformation, what the shoemaker has to attend to is the making of the necessary provision in the length, breadth, and other dimensions of the boot, to permit and accommodate the changes that are thus taking place in the foot.

245. In making the necessary provision in the construction of the boot just referred to, to accommodate the gradual restoration of the foot to its normal symmetry and beauty, many practical details are passed over that might, no doubt, be supplied; but they are so professional as to character, so dependent upon the individuality of every case, and at the same time so manifest, that it would be superfluous to notice them in a work of this kind. Attention has already been drawn to the stocking (115, 117, 118); and in the

improvement of injured toes, an easy well-fitting pair is the first desideratum required.*

* To prevent the stocking compressing the toes too much when forced into a close-fitting boot or shoe, a very useful and simple contrivance may be adopted : a blunt, pointed, flexible needle put through the toe of the stocking, across it, at about an inch from the extreme end ; to the needle is attached a tape, of sufficient length to allow the other end to remain outside the boot. When the foot is put into the boot, the needle is withdrawn by pulling the tape ; by this means the stocking is prevented from rucking at the heel, and the toes are free from any pressure of the stocking.

## CHAPTER XII.

ON TRADE SYSTEMS, AND THE COMPARATIVE MERITS AND CLAIMS OF THE ELASTIC PRINCIPLE.

246. In this chapter it is intended very briefly to notice the influence of what may be termed trade systems upon shoemaking under the following inquiries:—How far they have been instrumental in begetting and upholding the present objectionable style? What are the comparative merits of the elastic principle? What is the duty and interest of the public generally in the progress of this principle? And what are the objections to the use of elasticated leather, and other fabrics of this kind, now being introduced and extensively worn in every rank of society?

247. As to trade systems, boots and shoes are made to order, according to the measure of the person who gives the order; or they are made to supply a large wholesale and retail business in ready-made goods; or they are made to order, according to pattern. In each case, the contract may be large or small, from a single pair up to many thousands.

248. As to commercial value, a pair of Wellingtons, from a customer point of view, may cost

from 7s. 6d. to £2. and upwards; other kinds of boots and shoes being equally diversified as to price.

249. As to intrinsic value, differences are even greater than as regards the money-price of boots and shoes.

250. And as to style, generally speaking, there is something of a fashionable family likeness in all descriptions of boots and shoes, so to speak, all being equally liable to distort the foot (219).

251. There is nothing, therefore, that characterizes any one of the above systems more than the others of being responsible for present shortcomings. We must consequently endeavour to trace the present unpropitious state of things, as shown in a previous section (219), to a common source, and this will, no doubt, be found in a too limited knowledge of the physiological anatomy of the human foot, and the common tendency, on the part of St. Crispin and his last-maker, to make the most of the sweat of their brow, to meet the desire for low-priced goods.

252. We have here two sides of a great public question—the foot-dress of all classes of the community—to examine; and whatever may be said in extenuation of the past as regards either side, it is manifest that no excuse whatever can be pleaded for the continuation of the present style of boots and shoes. Indeed, such is the anomalous state of things, that Social Science has not even a single apology to

## ON TRADE SYSTEMS. 187

advance in their favour ; for, commercially, they are dear at any price—intrinsically, they are worth less than nothing ; while, as regards style, distorted feet, crooked toes, corns, bunions, *et id genus omne*, are, perhaps, the nearest estimation that can practically be given of their value.

253. We then come to the comparative merits of the elastic principle, with the consequential duties involved, and without stopping to make a single inquiry as to the peculiar position of the past in this respect, there cannot be a doubt but responsibilities are now very different from what they have been ; for by a timely and proper discharge of duty all may realize a real interest in advancing the cause of progress. This conclusion is manifest, whether examined from a pecuniary point of view, or purely from that of the physical wellbeing of the foot ; for we shall now proceed to prove to the reader that that which preserves the foot in health will be found at the same time the cheapest covering. In other words, an elastic waist introduced into the sole of the boot or shoe, will make it, not only more comfortable than the rigid-soled one, but also last longer, the increase in the length of time doing more than counterbalancing any extra expense in the manufacture, because the wearer in the case of the elastic sole walks with a lighter and less grinding step than in the case of the rigid sole, as has already been shown (161, 213, 230).

254. There are thus two advantages gained, each of which requires consideration, viz., the greater health and usefulness of the foot, and the greater durability of the boot, because both are involved in the question of pecuniary value, and in the general question of the best and cheapest covering for the foot.

255. It has already been shown, that the health, strength, and beauty of the human foot is susceptible of cultivation by proper means (68), and we now proceed to show that this has been known to all civilized nations in every age of the world. The attention paid by the ancient Greeks and Romans in their gymnasiums and other places to improve the muscular development and strength of their youth, especially of the arms, feet, and legs, in those aspiring to eminence in military life, must be familiar to every reader of history, as also the high value put upon such training by all classes of society, ancient and modern. In our own day, if gymnastic exercise is less practised generally among the masses of the people, it is not valued at a less estimate by our medical men; while we see in those engaged in the Spanish bull-fights, and in our own equestrian amphitheatres, what can be done in improving the muscular development and strength of the lower extremities. In all these cases, the practical question at issue, when reduced to its simplest form, is clearly the human foot in the highest degree of health, strength,

and beauty, and the means by which such important blessings are obtained—blessings now manifestly within the reach of all.

256. We have thus in these examples to attend to two important principles of a kindred character, or two simple means to obtain two important ends— viz., exercise to strengthen the foot, and elasticity to strengthen the boot ; and from such, as fundamental principles, we come to their reduction to practice, as involved in the general question, What are the duties and responsibilities which they involve ? What, for example, is the duty of parents and guardians, and of public institutions for the education and training of youth ? What is the duty of those in authority in the public service who control the supplying of our Army, Navy, and Police with boots and shoes ? Of those at the head of the Volunteer movement ? Of St. Crispin himself ?—of his last-maker ? And, in short, what is the duty of all who wear boots and shoes, individually and collectively ?

257. So unanimous is public opinion in favour of moderate exercise as an invaluable source of health, that its cultivation by such means must be acknowledged a public duty. And if this is true of the body as a whole, then the foot cannot be pleaded as an exception, especially since the general health is so dependent upon the physical well-being of the foot (59).

258. It is rather singular, however, that so little

attention should have hitherto been paid to the proper development of the foot of man by means of muscular exercise, especially considering the incredible amount of pain and suffering that is experienced by the contrary treatment, so generally exemplified in the derangement of its functions; and at the same time considering further, that so much attention should be paid to health-giving exercise in the shoeing of the horse, to restore the foot of that invaluable servant, when lamed, to a state of soundness.

259. The old maxim, that "prevention is better than cure," is a sound one. Taking this maxim, then, as our motto, the proposition that, if the amount of lameness now experienced amongst all classes, and in all ages, from injured and distorted feet, can be obviated by boots and shoes having elasticated leather introduced into certain parts, as was shown in the preceding chapter, it naturally follows, that such a desideratum should be generally realized, and that it will be so whenever the physiological anatomy of the foot, and the nature and comparative merits of such a covering are properly understood.

260. It is clearly, therefore, the duty of parents and guardians of youth, who, as such, have the privilege of thinking for so large a portion of the community, to make themselves thoroughly acquainted with the heavy responsibility under which

they lie. The soundness of this conclusion hardly admits of proof, as the subject is now one clearly open to their investigation, for the growth of crooked toes and "bachlin children" are becoming daily more and more incompatible with Social Science.

261. It is still more imperatively the duty of Government to study the best plan of shoeing a soldier. The best use of the lower extremities is, doubtless, a practical question in military science. It is now long since Marshal Saxe advocated low heels and thin flexible soles for the foot-gear of the French soldier, in order to give him the full faculty of his feet and legs (see foot-note, 93); and a public writer on the late war expresses a similar wish, in reference to the European force engaged by this country in India (foot-note, 93). In both cases, the conclusions are deduced from observations of the sufferings experienced by our troops in having to wear rigid, unbending leather, and the advantages gained by other troops, as the Sepoys, in the wear of thin shoes or sandals, allowing the foot the free and unrestrained use of its natural functions; and that the conclusions are sound in principle, and point to the necessity of a change in the shoeing of our soldiers, requires no further proof than has already been advanced (219) in a previous chapter.

262. Official management in this department of the Government is so highly reprehensible as to call

for practical exposure.* Such is the total disregard, or, perhaps, we should say, ignorance displayed relative to the functions and physical well-being of the soldier's foot, that all the most objectionable characteristics of the ordinary boots and shoes worn are selected as the cardinal qualifications of a regulation boot for the public service!—such, for example, as high heels, convex rigid waist, and turned-up, wedge-shaped toes—characteristics which have been shown pregnant with mischief to the health of the foot and the sanitary condition of the body generally. So incredible are the facts of the case experienced by the soldier when called upon active duty in time of war, that they must be seen to be believed (see foot-note 219). An army of soldiers marching under all the exciting elements of active hostilities in modern warfare is a very different affair from an individual on a journey, even if that should be in a hostile country; for if the latter becomes weakly, he can suit his step to his

---

* When attending Sir George Ballingall's Lectures on Military Surgery in the Edinburgh University, he, in lecturing on the clothing of the army, stated, "That it was much to be regretted that the medical officers of the army were not consulted respecting the soldier's clothing and boots; the greater part of which is ill adapted to the soldier's requirements, especially his boots," one of which he held in his hand, and drew the attention of his students to its shape and construction, with its convex sole and high heel; in contrast to the beautiful concave elastic arch of the foot of a skeleton, which was suspended from the ceiling of the lecture-room.

## ON TRADE SYSTEMS. 193

strength, and if he breaks down it is but an individual case. But in the march of large armies, when the weak are compelled to step out with the strong; and where lameness and its consequences are brought on by the rigid-soled regulation boots of the public service, then the system becomes a Juggernaut of cruelty, which only the carnage of a campaign in foreign lands can illustrate—every retreat and forced march under such circumstances being strewn with the carcases of footsore soldiers!*

263. It does not require logic to prove that the strength of an army depends upon the use it can make of its feet and legs, and that the recent improvements in firearms greatly increase the value of such qualifications. A soldier may be strong in the arms, but if lame or weak in his feet he can never apply with advantage the strength of his arm in charging the enemy with the bayonet, or in sustaining the charge of the enemy, simply because in both cases the foot is that part of the mechanical system of leverage (21, 197, 202, 203) that rests upon the fulcrum, the ground; so that if the leverage is weakened at this important point, the strength of the whole system is inevitably reduced. This is a well-known fact to Engineers, "Clerks of

---

* Gen. Sir Thomas Willshire told me he lost a considerable number of his men in the Affghan war by their becoming footsore, and consequently unable to keep up with the main body, when the enemy from the heights picked them off with the greatest ease.

Works," and all who have any experience as workmen, where the foot has to sustain the force applied; and the soldier is no exception to this rule; for, when footsore, he may thrash downwards with the but-end of his gun, but to charge with the point of the bayonet, or defend himself as he should do, is impossible. For a similar reason, the soldier, who is not footsore, is prevented by the rigid regulation-boot from putting forth his full force in charging the enemy or in defending himself. It is an experimental knowledge of this that makes our native soldiers of the Indies, West and East, throw aside their regulation-boots, forced upon them by our Government (see foot-note, 219). Even to order the soldier " *To stand at ease*" in the foot-gear of the public service is no less an insult to common sense than to humanity (188)!

264. On the contrary, as the medical department of the army rejects unsound feet, and only passes recruits who are sound (see foot-note, 237), let us now entertain the proposition of using foot-gear that will improve their feet after they enter the service, instead of injuring them, as we have seen is the case at present. If the Greeks and Romans of old were successful in their "military gymnasiums," in improving the muscular development of their soldiers, cannot we do the same by similar means? No doubt, the stimulus of light on the nude body will be so far against us, but otherwise, is it not possible to im-

prove upon their practice? If we adopt their practice in reference to the whole of the body save the foot and neck, as we already unquestionably do, why make two such important parts of the soldier an exception? If by a spring from his well-trained elastic foot the king of the forest brings the weight of his body into action in making a charge, can we not take a lesson from this example in the school of Nature? Let us, then, once more propose to take off the rigid regulation-boots from the pinched toes of the British soldier, and put on elastic ones, that will allow him the free exercise of his feet and legs, so essentially necessary to the rapid progression of modern warfare and an effective charge when he comes to close quarters. All this has been shown to be not more sound in theory than profitable in practice ; and if the cheapest system of shoeing the soldier is that which affords him the most comfort, and makes him the most effective when in the discharge of his duty, ought it not to be adopted?

265. In corroboration of the above, it may be mentioned to those readers not acquainted with the blue books on the public service, that experiments have been made with elastic boots in the army, and that results prove, beyond a doubt, that both the above conclusions can be realized ; viz., that the soldier can be more cheaply shod per annum, while his health, strength, and usefulness can be greatly increased.

266. What has just been said in reference to the soldier relative to the improvement of the muscular development, health, strength, and elastic qualifications of the lower extremities, is equally, if not more applicable, to the volunteer. After what has already been said in a previous section (73), it would be superfluous to impress upon the attention of those at the head of this national movement the importance of cultivating a more dignified step than the rocking lever one of our troops in the regular service. From long use and habit, we may not, at first sight, see the want of gracefulness in the amount of heel-work and knee-work exemplified in walking in rigid-soled boots, and the heavy sacrifice of muscular force thus sustained ; but by a very superficial investigation, these will readily become perceptible. Health is one of the most important realizations of the volunteer movement, and the gymnastic means for improving the symmetry and beauty of every member of the body should be studiously attended to. The movement, although it has a military aspect when superficially examined, is, nevertheless, when more closely investigated, one of the most important sanitary branches of Social Science.

267. With regard to the duty of shoemakers, last-makers, and the public generally, the common cause is the common interest. Fashion may have her votaries and her influence ; but the age in which we live is daily becoming more and more utilitarian in

character, and there cannot be a doubt but the present system—if system it can be called—of sacrificing the usefulness of the human foot is doomed; and that even Fashion herself, in spite of all the prejudices of the past, is about to "pack up her old traps," with a view to starting afresh on sounder principles in the shoeing of man. There is an old toast with which all are no doubt familiar:—

"Here's to our friends! As for our foes,·
May they have short shoes, and corns on their toes."

—the plain English of which is embodied in what a Prime Minister once told me in reply to something that fell from my lips, perhaps too much in favour of St. Crispin,—"Shoemakers should be all treated like pirates,—put to death without trial or mercy,—as they had inflicted more suffering on mankind than any class he knew." The above nobleman is well known for the precision with which he "hits the nail on the head;" and however reluctantly we may say it, there cannot be a doubt but "*a hobnail*" is here driven into St. Crispin's heel, that must be removed before he can "stand at ease."

268. With regard to objections to elasticated leather, and the principle it involves in the manufacture of boots and shoes, doubtless many can be raised; but they are as easily refuted. It has, for example, been said that "the elastic waist would not stand the spade in digging." Granted; but

neither does the rigid sole. Both require "a tramp," or "foot-iron." Digging with a spade, whether in agriculture, in horticulture, at railway-work, or in military trench-works, is an artificial application of the foot that requires special provision to protect the sole, and this provision is "a tramp," or "foot-iron." With such a provision, the foot with an elastic-waisted boot will do more work than with a rigid-soled one, because in the former case the muscular strength of the foot is greater. Rigid boots, by weakening the muscles, reduce the strength of the foot, and, consequently, the force applied to the rigid sole; and although this may be one way of making rigid soles stand the spade, as in military trench-work, it is certainly not a valid one, but the reverse; for the more scientific, practical, and successful plan of doing work is to increase the muscular power of the foot by an elastic covering, and then put on a strong foot-iron to stand the increase of force thus applied to the spade or other digging implement. The objection is thus worse than fallacious, and so are all others to the elastic principle.

## CHAPTER XIII.

### CONCLUDING REMARKS.

269. In the preceding chapters, the importance of the subject of the foot and its covering, however imperfectly treated, cannot fail to have arrested the reader's attention. Much in every age has been written on the shoeing of the horse and other domesticated animals by men of the highest rank in science and practice; but how much more worthy of scientific and experimental investigation is the best plan of shoeing man, considering the widely diversified circumstances he is called upon to experience, and the necessary protection his foot requires in every case.

270. When we look at the domestic habitations of the human race, we see a wide difference between the palace and the humble cottage by the wayside. When we turn to the citadel of the swallow in the corners of our windows, or to that of the sparrow in the hedge, we see a uniformity of design, and a common purpose served in every case. If we descend another step lower in the animal kingdom, we see creatures crawling about with their houses (shells) on their backs—citadels into which they creep for

protection; and so unique is the accommodation afforded, and so adapted in every case to the physical well-being of its owner, that no one has ever ventured to improve upon the original design of either the animal or the habitation provided for it by its Creator. In its covering there is no lack of room, but nothing over. It is Nature's work, and a " perfect fit."

271. Nature is truly instructive in all her works. *To this rule there is no exception;* and the above examples are not without their modicum of information to the shoemaker; for, in the first place, they draw his attention to the fact, that in an old house, or even in an old shoe, may be seen a faithful illustration of fallen humanity, and how far man in all his works is behind Nature; and in the second place, that to ply successfully his vocation as a shoemaker, in providing protection for the foot of man it is absolutely necessary to study closely those fundamental principles which Nature has established throughout all her works. In other words, he must make himself thoroughly acquainted with the anatomical mechanism of the human foot, simply because it is for this peculiar mechanism, in all its ever-varying positions, that he has to provide suitable accommodation and protection. Structurally and physiologically, the foot of man is a piece of exquisitely fine workmanship, admirably adapted for the purpose it serves in the animal economy; and the professional skill and artistic handicraft of the shoemaker

is illustrated by the covering he provides for its internal and external accommodation. Outwardly to appearance, standing in an erect attitude is a very simple affair, easily performed by a child, after a little experimental training, the philosophy of which is often thought little about. And yet, as Dr. Knox observes in his invaluable work on " Man, his Structure and Physiology," " to do so, an almost incredible number of muscles are called into action." The same takes place in walking. And, according to the author just quoted, so powerful are the muscles of the thigh, that "they not unfrequently snap the patella across." Now the strength of these and all the other muscles of the lower extremities must be preserved, and one of the fundamental laws already referred to, and essentially necessary to preserve muscles, tendons, ligaments, and bones in health and strength, *is exercise*. The shoemaker, therefore, must make suitable provision for the free and unrestrained action of the foot in all its movements.

272. The measurement, therefore, of the foot—an organism so beautiful in its symmetry, so wonderful in its mechanism, and with so important functions to perform—requires consummate skill on the part of the shoemaker; and to apply that measurement to the last, so as to turn out a proper fit of boots or shoes, capable of affording free play to the foot, as above (271), requires perhaps a still greater degree of professional talent; yet all this

must be done to provide for the internal wants of the foot, and at the same time to protect it from external injury.

273. How far the present construction of boots and shoes, generally speaking, makes provision for the functions of the foot, is our next inquiry; and under this division of our subject, it is much to be regretted that a more favourable report cannot be given. High heels, rigid soles curved downwards at the waist and upwards at the toes, and wedge-toed uppers, are altogether incompatible with the physiological anatomy of the human foot. There is, therefore, no alternative left but a sweeping condemnation against all incompatibles of this kind that metamorphose beautiful symmetry into ugly distortion—health-giving action into excruciating suffering and misery—the lower extremities, with all their elastic mechanical contrivances, into rigid rocking levers, and the graceful dignity of walking into an awkward jolting hobble, more easily imagined than described.

274. Lastly, the proposition of elasticating material for the construction of boots and shoes, the adaptation of such to the functions of the foot, its economy, and other questions of this kind, are discussed. The manufacture of fabrics possessing the property of expanding and contracting to accommodate the extension and contraction of the muscles, and also possessing pliant properties, adapted to the different flexions of the foot, is unquestionably sound

## CONCLUDING REMARKS. 203

in principle; for if the covering is properly made of such material, it will afford to all the muscles, tendons, ligaments and bones of the foot free play internally, and also the necessary protection externally—the two grand desiderata at issue—what may not inaptly be termed the shoemaker's problem. From a pecuniary or economical point of view, as well as from a physical, experience has pronounced her verdict in favour of this new movement in the clothing of the foot.

275. Such is the close of this little treatise. Supported by the concurring testimony of all that is necessary to aid in advancing the cause of progress, the subject advocated in its pages may with every degree of confidence be left to the dispassionate consideration of the reader. The protection and welfare of the human foot involves much to engage attention and stimulate inquiry relative to a knowledge of its beautiful mechanism and organization. How soon will its component elements be returned to the earth from whence they were taken! The foot of man is truly but a short-lived organism—generally the first on which the cold hand of death is laid; but while life remains, there is in every breast a law that demands the sanitary preservation of it and every other member of the body. How interesting is the study of the laws of nature thus implanted in the human breast. How beautiful is the harmony that exists between them and the greatest degree of health and happiness which the human frame can corpo-

really enjoy ; and how undeniable the evidence furnished by this *harmony* that HE who gave being to Nature's laws at first continues still to uphold them, thus wisely demanding the fealty of all HIS creatures for their own physical well-being. How anxious, therefore, should every one be to render obedience to these laws, in order to enjoy what can only thus be obtained, the inestimable blessing of " A LENGTH OF HAPPY DAYS."

THE END.

www.ingramcontent.com/pod-product-compliance
Lightning Source LLC
Chambersburg PA
CBHW020835160426
43192CB00007B/667